the

A FULL CIRCLE BOOK

the tao of reiki

A Transpersonal Pathway to an Ancient Healing Art

Including

Dr. Usui's original manuscripts, Reiki's Founding Father

By
Lawrence Ellyard

FULL CIRCLE

Medical Disclaimer

The methods presented here should by no means replace conventional medical practice or the advice prescribed by qualified health professionals. Reiki is seen as a complementary therapy to health care, but it is in no way a substitute or a replacement for conventional medical practice. In the case of serious medical or psychological illness, consult a qualified medical practitioner.

THE TAO OF REIKI

FULL CIRCLE

First Indian Paperback Edition, 2001
First revised edition, 2002
ISBN 81-7621-004-8

Published by **FULL CIRCLE**
18-19, Dilshad Garden, G.T. Road, Delhi-110 095
Tel: 228 2467, 229 7792 • Fax: 228 2332
e-mail: fullcircle@vsnl.com

Print & Production: SCANSET

18-19 Dilshad Garden, G.T. Road, Delhi-110 095
Tel: 228 2467, 229 7792 Fax: 228 2332

Printed at Nutech Photolithographers, Delhi-110 095

PRINTED IN INDIA

Contents

Foreword

When I first received the material by Dr. Usui from my father, and chose to begin the translation and utilization of the material, I seriously pondered the matter. Although at the time I knew nothing about Reiki other than a great deal of gossip and hearsay along with an earlier unfavorable impression, but being a Vajrayana Buddhist Lama I felt I knew something about Buddhism, and a bit about Japanese Buddhism, since I had grown up within the Shingon tradition.

I was in a quandary, should I read up on Reiki, familiarize myself with the systems, before tackling the material? However, after a great deal of thought and meditation, I chose to let Dr. Usui speak directly to me, one Buddhist to another, through his writings. I have not regretted that decision, in fact, I am feeling much relieved that I followed my first instincts.

In the last year I have read a number of books on Reiki of one kind or another, and was not only confused but disappointed. I have talked to a number of Masters of different systems and am amazed at the variety of practices and opinions. That is not to say I disagree or disparage those books in any way, but as the Buddha himself said, "All teachings are of the nature of the absolute arising of truth."

Now for some reason, Dr. Usui is somewhat shrouded in mystery, and in my readings, and my discussions with other Masters and practitioners, I have encountered a truly divergent mass of material. One story about Dr. Usui I have to discount as somewhat fabulous, as the same story was told about the Kobo Daishi (circa 805 AD), but this sort of thing is not uncommon about great and famous men. Since very little of our material is dated and in no way chronologically organized, we have a few glimpses into Usui's life, but not set out in any chronological order. When either Dr. Usui, or perhaps Dr. Wantanabe, we do not know which, organized the material, it was not organized in a chronological manner, but roughly indexed according to level of teaching and subject matter.

One section, for example, contained material which according to its contents could be dated 1890, 1900, or 1919. Trying to be an objective scholar and not a fastidious meddler, I have made no attempt to place my own chronology on the material. This I have left for others to do, and I believe Lawrence Ellyard's book, for which I am writing this foreword, does exactly that.

Lawrence casts new light on the life of Dr. Usui, for which any practitioner of Reiki should be consummately grateful. After reading his manuscript, I was amazed at the amount of material he had acquired. The logical and precise way he had arranged it and the depth of scholarship which went into his endeavor, present to me an overview which threw a great deal of light on much of my material. I was also able to then understand some of the time frame of the material with which I was working and even perceive a definite pattern of the evolution of the system in Dr. Usui's own mind.

The book is lucid, concise, exceedingly rational and immanently readable. The presentation shows profound scholarship as well as a clear understanding of the material presented. I can heartily recommend this scholastic work to all of my Men Chhos Reiki students, as well as to all of those who are practicing any form for Dr. Usui's system of Reiki. I am sure that his book in the future will serve as a true reference volume and I truly consider it to be the definitive work to date on Dr. Usui's life and practice.

Lama Yeshe
(Dr. Richard Blackwell)
Winston-Salem, NC
August 2000

Preface

The information presented within this book should in no way replace the direct transmission required from a qualified Reiki teacher. To become a Reiki practitioner requires a living teacher, who is empowered to facilitate the correct initiations in the original Reiki lineage.

The methods presented here are a guide to anyone who is considering learning Reiki or, for established practitioners and teachers who wish to develop a wider understanding of Reiki and its applications.

This book does not attempt to convey or describe the empowerments required to facilitate the Reiki system. It is, however, a guide to support a Reiki practitioner or Reiki teacher's practice in the Western Reiki System.

Author's Note

This book was written as a guide to share traditional methods, as well as introduce the reader to the broad spectrum of Reiki, and its myriad of expressions and forms. The content of this book is by no means the final word on the practice of Reiki. The methods presented are a collective of my experiences and training received in both Western and Eastern Reiki systems.

Documents from Dr. Usui's manuscripts have been included in this text to present the reader with insight into the historical legitimacy of the Buddhist origins of Reiki healing, and to offer a window into the life and times of the founding father of Reiki. This material has kindly been made available by the Venerable Lama Yeshe and FULL CIRCLE. It is my hope that what little knowledge I possess of Reiki, be shared with the reader to hopefully spark some personal insight and healing, so that this in turn, may be shared with others.

Included in Section I are some excerpts from Dr. Usui's manuscripts. These manuscripts have received minimal adjustments in order to preserve an authentic presentation of Dr. Usui's teachings and views of Reiki.

The information presented within Section II of this

volume, outlines techniques and procedures in the Western Reiki system. The actual methodology of Medicine Dharma Reiki is not presented in this book, however it has been introduced as a means to educate the Reiki practitioner in the origins of Medicine Dharma Reiki as taught by Dr. Mikao Usui.

Since the first edition, I have received an overwhelmingly positive response to the material presented. With the continued research of Dr. Usui's manuals and the challenges which arises in translation, you may encounter when making comparison to the first edition, some minor changes. Some of which include historical updates as well as further authentication of the Reiki History.

The book's title has also generated some enquiry, regarding why I chose the title, the Tao of Reiki. This is by no means intended to draw a parallel between Reiki and Taoist belief. The word 'Tao', roughly translates as 'the way' and refers simply in this case, as the 'Way' of Reiki. I sincerely hope that you will enjoy this revised edition and may it serve you as a thought provoking guide to the practice of Reiki.

Lawrence Ellyard
Fremantle, Western Australia, April 2002.

Dedication

For the benefit of all that lives.

SECTION ONE

History of Reiki

Chapter 1

'We are all joined together by the chain that is Life on this planet, and to us Life should be precious and a unity.'
— ***Mikao Usui****, Reiki's Founding Father*

HISTORY OF REIKI

The healing art of Reiki, like many healing traditions, is an active vehicle to heal the body, spirit and mind. It is a gentle way to bring back the disconnected parts of self and to reawaken an ancient part of the healing mind. Although these teachings are new to the West, the origins of Reiki stretch back to ancient times, where this healing force, this gift from the ancients, was kept, only to a select few.

In Western terms, this healing art is still a newborn in light of its long and distant past.

The spiritual method to assist humanity in finding their humanity. However, the origins of Reiki throughout time have been clouded in mystery, uncertainty and oftentimes, speculation.

Facts concerning Reiki's founder, Dr. Mikao Usui and the details of his life path have remained unclear, as no physical records were kept of his life and his system of healing. A student, of the west, or teacher for that matter, has had to rely on the Reiki 'oral' tradition, which over time has become more likened to a great 'Chinese Whisper'. As Reiki was passed from one teacher to the next, this oral tradition, became more and more misrepresented and distorted, leaving the Reiki teachings, somewhat altered from their original form.

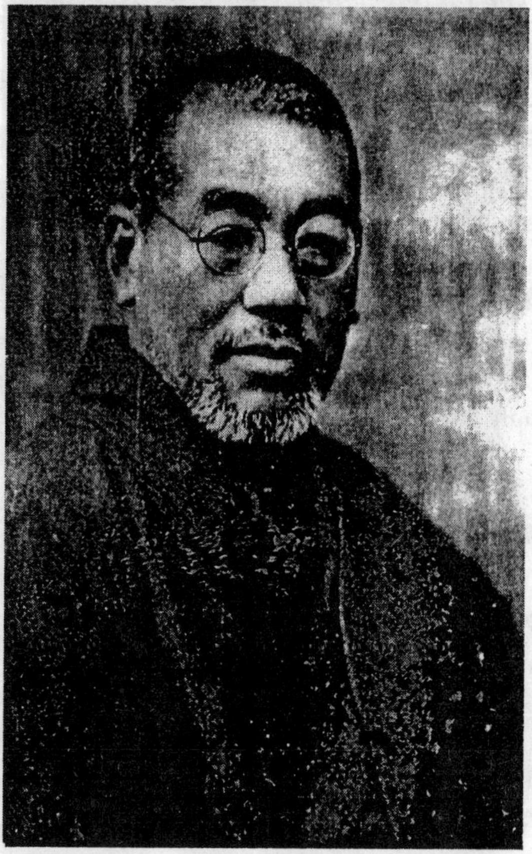

Dr. Usui
(Used with kind permission of Phyllis Lei Furumoto.)

The history of Reiki was faced with the fate of fading into myth or legend, until the recent discovery of the lost teachings of the Reiki System.

Dr. Usui's teachings, discovered in 1994, were unearthed to finally detail the exact history and precise science of this ancient healing art. These manuscripts detail the life and times of Reiki's founder, the historical verification of Reiki's roots, and the complete and intact Reiki healing tradition.

Fortunately, with the discovery of Dr. Usui's manuscripts, much of the oral transmission and teachings have now come to light. With this new information, comes a deeper validity to the Reiki system which in turn adds a solid foundation to the practices and methods of Reiki which spawned in Japan over a century ago.

THE LIFE STORY OF DR. MIKAO USUI – REIKI'S FOUNDING FATHER

This following account was written and compiled by the author and Gejong Palmo, a practitioner of Tibetan Buddhism. The content of this information extends to a variety of sources including facts derived from Usui's original manuscripts. This article captures the essence of the historical sequence of events of Usui's path and the developments, which proceeded until his death in 1926.

Mikao Usui was born in the village of Yago in the Gifu Prefecture on August 15, 1865, where his ancestors had lived for eleven generations. His family belonged to the Tendai sect of Buddhism. When he was four, he was sent to a Tendai Monastery to receive his primary education. He was a good student and was very bright.

Usui pursued higher education and received a doctorate in literature. He spoke many languages and became well-versed in medicine, theology and philosophy. Like many intellectuals of his day, Usui was fascinated with the 'new science' coming from the West. During this time (1880s and 90s), the Meiji Emperor had begun a new regime that overthrew the Shoguns and Japan's feudal states, now relocated in Tokyo, and were brought under the direct control of the central government. Under this new regime, the 'old ideas' were discarded in favour of modernization and the country was opened to westerners for the first time. There rose frenzy for transforming the modes of daily life into occidental fashions, which were identified with civilization. In every department of social and political life, men furnished with some knowledge of modern science were promoted to high positions. Men of 'new knowledge' were almost idolized and the ambition of every young man was to read the 'horizontal writings' of occidental books. The nation as a whole asked eagerly for the benefits of the new civilization. The motto of the era was 'Enlightenment and Civilization'.

Usui's father, Uzaemon, was an avid follower of the new regime and adopted progressive political views. Usui had great respect for his father and was very influenced by this national obsession to become 'westernized'. Usui continued to study science and medicine. In addition he befriended several Christian missionaries who had studied medicine at Harvard and Yale.

During this time when Japan was opening its doors to the West, the first arrivals were the missionaries, both Catholic and Protestant. They set up their operations in three main areas. One was in Yokohama, under the influence of Rev. John Ballagh. Here they started their medical work and brought with them knowledge of western medical science. These missionaries became very influential leaders and formed the first Japanese Christian church in 1872.

Throughout Usui's early adulthood, he lived in Kyoto with his wife, Sadako Sizuki, and two children, a son and a daughter. He was a businessman and had varying degrees of success. Usui did encounter some difficulties, but his strong determination and positive outlook on life helped him to overcome all obstacles. He continued his religious study and became involved with a group named 'Rei Jyutsu Ka'. This group had a centre at the base of the holy mountain, Kurama Yama, north of Kyoto. There is an ancient Buddhist temple, Kurama-dera on the 1,700 ft mountain which has a large statue of Amida Buddha and houses many artefacts that are part of the National Treasure. Built in 770 AD, the temple belonged to the Tendai sect of esoteric Buddhism. By 1945 the temple had evolved into an independent Buddhist sect. For centuries, Kurama Yama has been regarded as a power spot and many famous sages, as well as Emperors, go there to pray. The temple and surrounding areas are kept in their natural state and the mountain itself is the spiritual symbol of Kurama temple. Steps lead down to the base where one can sit and meditate. Nearby is a waterfall. Usui went to this area frequently to meditate.

It was during this time (1888) that Usui contracted Cholera as an epidemic swept through Kyoto. He had a profound near death experience in which he received visions of Mahavairochana Buddha and received direct instructions from him. This was a life changing experience for Usui that caused him to make a major reassessment of his life. He developed a keen interest in the esoteric science of healing as taught by Buddha, and he developed the compassionate wish that he may learn these methods in order to benefit mankind. When Usui recovered from his near fatal illness, he began to discuss his experiences with his family and family priest. They were outraged at his claims of seeing enlightened deities and the Tendai priest beat him over the head and chased him out of the Temple.

Determined to find the answers to his questions about this vision, Usui eventually met a Shingon Bonze, Watanabe Senior, who recognized Usui's tremendous spiritual potential and took him on as a student. Usui then became a devout Shingon Buddhist, which outraged his family even more and they removed him from the family ancestry. Usui was seen as a traitor to his family and ancestors. To this day, relatives refuse to talk about him, saying that it is against the will of their ancestors to speak his name. Even his daughter wrote a clause in her will that her father's name should never be spoken in her home.

Mikao Usui spent much time and money pursuing his new found spiritual path by studying and collecting Buddhist scriptures. In particular, he studied Buddhist healing techniques and invested an enormous amount of money collecting old medical texts. Usui had good political and academic connections and had many contacts in various countries searching for texts. For example, in Bombay, India, merchants travelling along the silk route through Tibet to China were given gold to find secret Buddhist healing texts. Usui was particularly interested in obtaining texts from Tibet.

Kyoto was home to many large and extensive Buddhist libraries and monasteries that had collections of ancient texts. Usui did much of his research there. For many years, Usui continued to collect, study and practice these medical texts. He became an advanced practitioner and meditation master. His closest friend, Watanabe Kioshi Itami, the son of his Buddhist teacher, became his most devout student. Over time, Usui became a respected and learned Buddhist teacher with a following of devoted students. They met regularly and Usui would teach from the texts that he had been collecting. The focus of his teachings was on healing and benefiting humankind through healing. They practiced elaborate rituals for averting newly created diseases that were ravaging Japan, as well as esoteric practices for healing every type of illness.

Mikao Usui was truly a man ahead of his time. He went against the social norms of his day, which were very sectarian and class oriented. Usui believed that everyone should have access to the Buddhist healing methods, regardless of religious beliefs. He wanted to find a way to offer these powerful methods to the common man, with no need for long, arduous practice. Out of his great compassion and determination, he vowed that he would some day find a way to develop a healing that would cure every type of disease and could be taught to anyone, regardless of background, education or religious beliefs.

It was during the late 1890s that Usui came in contact with a box containing manuscripts which turned out to be the methods he had sought for so many years. Therein lay the Tantra of the Lightning Flash, the secret transmission for healing all illnesses of body, speech and mind. This tantra provided information that he had been looking for and presented a comprehensive healing method derived from esoteric Buddhism as practiced in Tibet. The text dated back to the 7th Century and was brought to Japan by Kobo Daishi, the founder of Shingon Buddhism. Current research determines the Tantra holds a direct lineage to the Historical Buddha (563-480 BC).

Dr. Usui went to Mt. Kurama Yama (a holy mountain in Japan) on a short retreat to contemplate this material, to review the miraculous healing from his illness and to discover why it was he who had received the Medicine Tantra. At the completion of his time on Kurama Yama he gained an understanding of these methods and received insight into these Buddhist practices. After much contemplation and careful consideration he decided to share these teachings with others. Through the distillation of years of study and practice, Usui was able to perceive a method for bringing the essence of these Buddhist practices to the masses. Usui called this healing method 'Rei Ki'.

Usui first practiced his newly discovered method on his family and friends. Then he began to offer this healing method to the lower class district of Kyoto.

Kyoto is a religious centre and the people in the streets are taken in and cared for with each family looking out for its own. Usui opened his home to many and for seven years he brought Reiki to them. This gave him the opportunity to perfect and refine his new healing method. Meanwhile, he continued to hold regular classes for his growing 'circle' of Buddhist followers, and further developed and refined his system.

In 1921, Usui moved to Tokyo where he worked as the secretary to Pei Gotoushin, the Prime Minister of Tokyo. He opened a Reiki clinic in Harajuku, outside Tokyo and began to set up classes and teach his system of Reiki. Some of his foremost students, who received the teachings, include:

- Watanabe Kioshi Itami, his long time friend and student from Kyoto. It was Watanabe who inherited all of Usui's notes and the collection of Buddhist Tantras when Usui died;
- Taketomi, who was a naval officer;
- Wanami;
- Five Buddhist nuns; and
- Kozo Ogawa. Ogawa opened a Reiki clinic in Shizuoka City. He was very active in the administration of the Reiki society. He passed on his work to his relative, Fumio Ogawa, who is still alive today.

In 1922, Usui founded the Reiki society, called Usui Reiki Ryoho Gakkai, and acted as its first president. This society was open to those who had studied Usui's Reiki. This society still exists today and there have been six presidents since Usui:

Mr. Jusaburo Ushida 1865-1935,

Mr. Kanichi Taketomi 1878-1960,

Mr. Yoshiharu Watanabe (? - 1960),

Mr. Hoichi Wanami 1883-1975,

Ms. Kimiko Koyama 1906-1999,

and the current president Mr. Masayoshi Kondo.

This society started a new 'religion', or spiritual organization, which was a common practice at this time in Japan.

On September 1, 1923 the devastating Kanto earthquake struck Tokyo and surrounding areas. Most of the central part of Tokyo was levelled and totally destroyed by fire. Over 140,000 people were killed. In one instance, 40,000 people were incinerated to death when a fire tornado swept across the open area where they had sought safety. These fires were started when the quake hit at midday, when countless hibachi charcoal grills were ready to cook lunch. The wood houses quickly ignited as they collapsed from the tremors. Three million homes were destroyed leaving countless homeless. Over 50,000 people suffered serious injuries. The public water and sewage systems were destroyed and it took years for rebuilding to take place.

In response to this catastrophe, Usui and his students offered Reiki to countless victims. His clinic soon became too small to handle the throng of patients, so in February of 1924, he built a new clinic in Nakano, outside Tokyo. His fame spread quickly all over Japan and he began receiving invitations from all over the country to come and teach his healing methods. Usui was awarded a Kun

San To from the Emperor, which is a very high award (much like an honorary doctorate), given to those who have done honourable work. His fame soon spread throughout the region and many prominent healers and physicians began requesting teachings from him.

Just prior to this devastating earthquake in 1923, Usui had begun teaching a simplified form of Reiki to the public in order to meet increasing demand. Usui saw that his method of healing had tremendous potential for all people, so out of compassion to aid all sentient beings, he developed a non-religious Reiki form to suit them. This form is the foundation of what is now known as Western Reiki. Two of his most notable students included:

- Toshihiro Eguchi, who studied with Usui in 1923. Eguchi was the most prominent of his students who reportedly taught thousands of students before the war. It is largely through Eguchi that Reiki has continued on in Japan; and
- Chujiro Hayashi, who studied with Usui from 1922. Hayashi was one of the first of Usui's non-Buddhist students. Hayashi was a Methodist Christian, had very strong beliefs, and was not open to the esoteric nature of what Usui was teaching. Usui eventually sent Hayashi on his way. Hayashi used the knowledge learned from Usui to open a clinic in Tokyo. He replaced some of the format of Usui's teachings and created a system of 'degrees'. He also developed a more complex set of hand positions suitable for clinic use. Hayashi's clinic employed a method of healing that required several practitioners to work on one

client at the same time to maximize the energy flow. One way Hayashi encouraged practitioners to his clinic was to give Level first empowerments in return for a three month commitment as unpaid help. After this time he would offer the better students the second Level in return for a further nine month commitment. Those who completed this had the chance of receiving the Master symbol or third degree. After two years further commitment (which involved assisting Hayashi in the classroom), practitioners were taught the empowerments and were allowed to teach. No money exchanged hands in this training – practitioners simply had to work an eight hour shift once a week for the duration of the commitment. Hayashi subsequently passed his knowledge to Mrs. Takata, who was responsible for bringing Reiki to America in the 1970s. It should be stressed that the actual content of the Reiki system known in the West today bears but a fragment of Usui's actual Reiki system. Usui taught a simplified form of Reiki to Hayashi and in turn, Hayashi introduced new elements and structures to the Reiki system. Further to this, Mrs. Takata changed and added new material again to the system. So when Reiki finally came to the West, the Usui system had changed quite significantly and bore little resemblance to its former roots.

Usui quickly became very busy as requests for teachings of Reiki continued to grow. He travelled throughout Japan (not an easy undertaking in those days), to teach and give Reiki empowerments. This started to take its toll on his health and he began

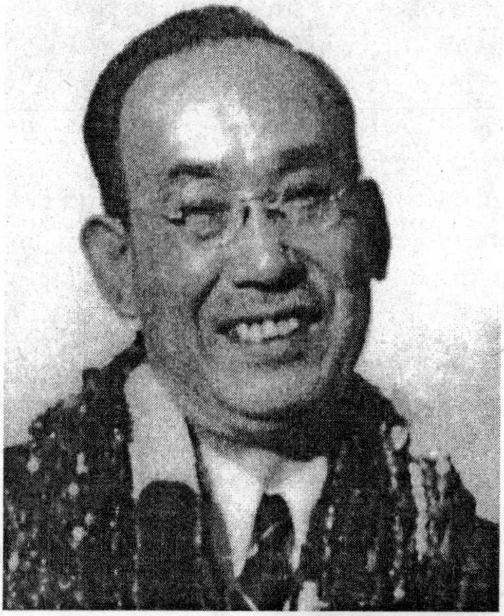

Mr. Hayashi

Mrs. Takata

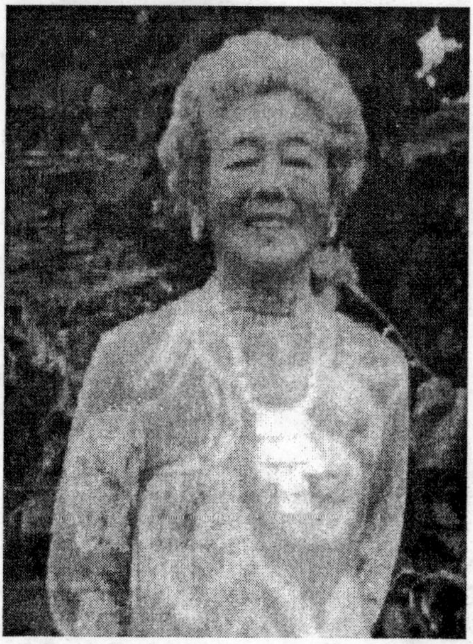

(Both the photographs used with kind permission of Phyllis Lei Furumoto)

experiencing mini-strokes from stress. Usui knew that he would soon die. One day, while in his office in Tokyo, he gathered all of his documents and materials on Reiki. All his class notes, his diary and the collection of sacred Buddhist texts were placed in a large lacquered box. He gave this to Watanabe, whom he considered his foremost student and dearest friend. Usui then left for a teaching tour in the Western part of Japan. Finally, on March 9, 1926, while in Fukuyama, Usui died of a fatal stroke. He was 62 years old.

Usui's body was cremated and his ashes were placed in a temple in Tokyo. Shortly after his death, students from the Reiki society in Tokyo erected a memorial stone at Saihoji Temple in the Toyatama district in Tokyo. According to the inscription on his memorial stone, Usui taught Reiki to over 2,000 people. However, as written in Dr. Usui's personal notes, he clearly states that he had taught over 700 students. Perhaps the students who erected his memorial stone mentioned 2,000 to praise Dr. Usui's teaching efforts. Many of these students began their own clinics and founded Reiki schools and societies. By the 1940s there were about 40 Reiki schools spread all over Japan. Most of these schools taught the simplified method of Reiki that Usui had developed. Another more secret Reiki Society continued to maintain the esoteric tradition. These practitioners did not bring their work out to the public and upheld a deeply spiritual basis for their work. It is unlikely that many westerners have encountered this faction of the Reiki teachings in Japan.

THE DISCOVERY OF THE ORIGINAL TEACHINGS IN THE WEST

Before Usui died, he passed the entirety of the Reiki system to his principal student and friend, Dr. Watanabe Kioshi Itami. In 1936, just prior to Japan's involvement in World War II, Dr. Watanabe placed the notes and documents of the Tantra, along with Usui's manuscripts, in a small monastery in the northern Prefecture of Tokyo. The contents of the Tantra and other documents remained in the original black lacquered box. Knowing he was going to be out of the country, Watanabe left the documents at the monastery. (It was a common practice in Japan to put one's documents in a monastery for safe keeping; it was similar in function to a safety deposit box in banks today.)

Dr. Watanabe was drafted in 1942 and subsequently died in the battle between Japan and the American forces in Manila, Philippines in 1944. The monastery where the texts were kept was also fire bombed during the war. The black box and the documents were saved from the fire bombing when they were carried out to the park surrounding the monastery, by the resident monks. Shortly after the war, the Buddhist monks began touring other temples, taking with them old manuscripts, including the Tantra of the Lightning Flash and Usui's complete Reiki system. They were looking to sell these texts, in order to generate the necessary funds to rebuild their monastery. The monks who were in possession of these texts were of little scholarly education and did not realize the content of the teachings they were going to sell. In 1946 these monks visited a Shingon temple where at the time, an American Army officer (Captain Blackwell) was receiving instruction in Shingon Buddhism. The monks in residence had themselves no money to offer, so Captain Blackwell offered to purchase these manuscripts from the monks. Giving them what he could, Captain Blackwell purchased the black lacquered box containing the Reiki System, he himself not knowing what he held in his hands. Captain Blackwell was deeply interested in the Japanese Buddhist traditions and wanted to help these monks as best he could.

One year later, Captain Blackwell and his wife had their first-born son in Yokohama, Japan. A further five years later, upon his return to the United States, Captain Blackwell decided to place these documents in storage in a safety deposit box in the Washington D.C. area. He decided that these texts may have some value, as they appeared very old, yet were in very good condition. As he did not speak the language written on the parchments, he had the title pages roughly translated. They translated describing spiritual healing methods with the words Rei Ki appearing repeatedly.

Captain Blackwell's son, Richard, grew up as a Shingon Buddhist, travelling around the world with his family. With such a strong Buddhist influence, Richard Blackwell developed a natural interest in Buddhist theology. When he was older, he studied Clinical Psychology and was employed at the National Institute for Mental Health. Interspersed with these activities, Dr. Richard Blackwell returned a number of times to Kathmandu and Nepal, receiving instruction in Buddhism. He was subsequently recognized as an incarnate Lama and took a traditional Lama retreat in Mustang, near the Tibetan border. In 1986

Dr. Richard Blackwell was ordained as Lama Yeshe Drugpa Trinley Odzer, the Ninth Drugmar Rinpoche of the Drugpa Kagyu Order of Bhutan.

Lama Yeshe then continued the life of a Lama, giving Buddhist teachings and instruction in the Dharma traditions. In 1994, Lama Yeshe (Dr. Richard Blackwell) rented a house in Portland, Oregon with his chief student, who was also a Reiki practitioner. One day, Lama Yeshe was speaking on the phone to his father in Brussels and casually mentioned his students Reiki activities. General Blackwell then remembered the texts he had purchased so long ago and, as a result of their conversation, Lama Yeshe began the arduous and slow process of having these texts translated. A German antiquarian later confirmed these as authentic manuscripts from the 7th to the 19th Century, detailing the Reiki tradition and teachings.

Lama Yeshe is an accomplished Buddhist master both in Bhutan, Tibetan and Shingon traditions. As these teachings are being translated, Lama Yeshe and initiated members of the Menchhos (Medicine Dharma) Reiki Sangha are transmitting these traditions among Buddhist and Reiki practitioners in a manner Usui would have done with his own students.

HISTORICAL FACTS – REIKI'S CHRONOLOGY

BC

563 Shakyamuni Buddha is born.
(During his teachings Buddha transmits the Lightning Flash Tantra to Ratnagharba.)

480	Shakyamuni Buddha dies.
	(The Lightning Flash Tantra is passed from Teacher to Disciple throughout India and China.)
AD	
774	Kobo Daishi is born.
805-810	Kobo Daishi establishes Shingon Buddhism in Japan, bringing the 'Tantra of the Lightning Flash'.
835	Kobo Daishi dies.
1865	Usui is born on August 15th in the first year of the Keio period.
1879	Chujiro Hayashi is born.
1880s	Usui completes Allopathic medical training.
1888	Usui contracts Cholera and experiences visions of Mahavairochana.
1899	Usui actualizes Reiki and begins teaching Reiki's Buddhist form.
1900	Mrs. Takata is born.
CA 1902-03	Usui opens his first Reiki Clinic in his home near Osaka.
1921	Usui opens second Reiki clinic in Harajuku, Tokyo.
1922	Usui founds the Reiki society: 'Usui Reiki Ryoho Gakkai'.
1923	Earthquake devastates Tokyo.
CA 1923-25	Usui starts teaching the simplified form of Reiki in order to meet public demand.
1924	Usui establishes new clinic outside Tokyo in Nakano.
1925	Chujiro Hayashi begins studying with Usui.
1925	Usui passes all his teachings and notes to his foremost student Watanabe.
1926	Usui dies of a fatal stroke on March 9, aged 62.
1926	Students of the Usui Reiki Ryoho Gakkai erect a memorial stone for Usui at Saihoji temple in the Toyotama district of Tokyo.
1930s	Hayashi establishes a clinic in Tokyo.

1936	Hayashi brings Reiki from Japan to the West when he visits Hawaii.
1936	Mrs. Takata learns Reiki from Hayashi.
1938	Mrs. Takata receives the complete empowerments for teaching Reiki.
1940	Mrs. Takata is declared as Hayashi's successor in his Reiki lineage.
1940	Chujiro Hayashi dies on May 10th.
1944	Dr. Watanabe dies in World War II.
1946	Captain Blackwell purchases the black lacquered box containing the 'Lightning Flash Tantra' and Usui's original manuscripts.
1970s	Mrs. Takata begins teaching Reiki in the United States of America and over a ten year period, initiates 22 students to teacher level.
1980	Mrs. Takata dies (Western Universal Reiki begins to be disseminated through the world).
1986	Dr. Richard Blackwell is recognized as a 'Tulku' and is ordained as the Venerable Lama Drugpa Yeshe Trinley Odzer, the Ninth Drumpar Rinpoche.
1994	Lama Yeshe discovers his father's manuscripts (Usui's system). A German antiquarian authenticates Usui's manuscripts and the Tantra of the Lightning Flash.
1994	Captain Blackwell's son, Lama Yeshe, receives the lacquered box and begins translations.
1995	Lama Yeshe begins teaching and giving empowerments in Usui's original teachings of Medicine Dharma Reiki (Menchhos Reiki).

MENCHHOS REIKI (MEDICINE DHARMA REIKI)

Menchhos Reiki, (pronounced 'Men-cho'), is the name given to the actual Buddhist form of Reiki that Usui taught prolifically in Japan before his death in 1926.

Lama Yeshe Trinley Odzer, the Ninth Drugmar Rinpoche, gave the name to the system to convey the meaning of this sacred medicine teaching. Since much of the material derived from Usui's original manuscripts is of early Indian Mahayana and Vajrayana origin, the material was given a Tibetan name. The meaning of 'Menchhos' is broken into two parts; Men — medicine or healing, and Chhos — supreme teaching or Dharma.

Essentially, Menchhos Reiki is largely derived from the Indian, Tibetan and Shingon Buddhist traditions. It is a hands on healing system with the direct transmission coming from the emanation of Medicine Buddha or 'Yakushi', in Japan. Medicine Buddha is the supreme Buddha of healing and, when properly invoked, can grant supernatural healing and empower the practitioner to propagate these healing works on the physical plane.

The Origins of Medicine Dharma Reiki (Usui's Reiki System)

Historical research derived from Dr. Usui's notes has determined that the origins of Reiki date back to Shakyamuni Buddha, the historical Buddha (563-480 BC). During his teaching career, which spanned some 50 years, Shakyamuni spoke the Sutra of Medicine Buddha, the Lord of the Lapis Lazuli Light (the Buddhist archetype for Healing). This teaching was passed from Shakyamuni to a physician known as 'Ratnagharba, the Womb of all Jewels'. The teaching passed to Ratnagharba was known as the 'Tantra of the Lightning Flash'. Throughout time, this healing tantra was passed from teacher to disciple in an unbroken lineage for over a thousand years. During this time, it made the journey across central Asia from India, Tibet and China, and finally to Japan in the 7th Century by the great Buddhist master, Kobo Dashi. These teachings were handed down throughout time from master to disciple, until they made their way to a Buddhist monastery in Hokkaido, Japan. Here these teachings stayed untouched by human hand for some three hundred years.

As the Buddhist monks in residence were of little education and did not know how to apply these teachings, whilst undertaking renovations of their monastery, they sold these texts to a book dealer who was touring the area looking for interesting volumes. The book dealer later carried these texts to Kyoto and it was here that Mikao Usui came into contact with these teachings. Soon after, Usui began studying these sacred texts with his Buddhist master, Watanabe Senior. It was after much diligence and practice that Usui began to grasp the essential teachings of the Tantra. These teachings laid the foundation to the development of Dr. Usui's Reiki system, which was strongly influenced by Vajrayana Buddhism and the Shingon Buddhist tradition.

How does Western Reiki and Usui's Dharma Reiki differ?

Medicine Dharma Reiki (Menchhos Reiki, Usui's Dharma Reiki), was the original Reiki system that incorporated the Buddhist tantras and empowerments derived from the 'Lightning Flash Tantra' and Usui's methods.

The Universal Reiki system, which has flourished in

the West as a direct result of Takata's teachings, is but a simplified portion of the complete Reiki teachings. Chujiro Hayashi, who was one of Usui's students, taught Universal Reiki to Mrs. Takata. Usui sought to teach a form of Reiki which was for everyone, regardless of religious beliefs, and in the last year of his life, Hayashi was taken on as a student in this non-Buddhist simplified form of Reiki. Universal Reiki, which comes from the lineage of Hayashi and Takata, is the familiar form which most western practitioners have in part and very few hold intact today. However, this form is vastly different to Usui's original system.

Today, many western teachers describe traditional Western Reiki as the 'Usui System of Natural Healing' and there had been many attempts at copyrighting the 'Usui' name. However, in light of this new information, and looking at the actual origins and developments of the Reiki system, it is clear that the original Usui System of Natural Healing bears little or no resemblance to Western Reiki. The western system would be better represented as the Hayashi/Takata Reiki system. In the last twenty years, Reiki in the West has taken many new forms. With the development of many new Western Reiki systems, there has been a number of changes to what is referred to as the Usui System of Natural Healing. For example, names like Sekhem, Seichim, Karuna, Tera-Mai, Johre, Raku-Reiki, Tibetan Reiki, and other recent Reiki developments, would be best described as non-traditional Reiki systems. These systems have largely been adapted and derived from Traditional Western Reiki, channelled information and other esoteric traditions. Many of these new Reiki systems are widely advertized on the internet. To avoid confusion for the reader, these other Reiki systems have been mentioned. Over the years, I have encountered many new forms of the Western Reiki system, and even more confusion amongst students who are often somewhat baffled with all the Reiki styles available. With so many variations on the market, it is hard to know where and from whom to learn Reiki. If you have an interest in non-traditional Reiki forms, I recommend learning traditional Western Reiki from a reputable teacher, who is empowered to pass on the tradition. Once a firm foundation has been established in traditional Reiki, explore till your heart's content. These new Reiki systems certainly have their place as healing modalities and now many Reiki teachers make clear distinctions between traditional and non-traditional Reiki forms.

The content within section two of this book attempts to describe the actual practices of the traditional Western Reiki system. Some additional practices which support and extend beyond the traditional system have also been included, for example, in Chapter 16 on Advanced Reiki.

Universal Reiki is a very 'user-friendly' healing system. One does not need any specific requirements to learn this system, as the methods taught do not align with any particular religious or a specific spiritual background.

When examining Medicine Dharma Reiki, it is clearly a more complex system. Aligning itself more closely to Vajrayana Buddhist Arising Yoga, and with some similar parallels to Central Asian Shamanism.

Medicine Dharma Reiki has a greater emphasis on

spiritual development and dedication on behalf of the student. To receive the original transmissions in Medicine Dharma Reiki, a student requires Buddhist refuge and is encouraged to embrace an understanding of the base concepts of Buddha Dharma practice.

In honouring the original Reiki system as it stands today, one can only qualify to receive these teachings in this way. The material contained within the Tantra is a complete healing system according to traditional Buddhist methodology. It is for these reasons why one needs to be qualified to receive initiation. Menchhos Reiki students are generally screened to discern their personal motivation and intentions before they are allowed to learn from the Sensei. This is not from exclusive or sectarian views, it is simply a matter of qualification and generating the right motivation. For Menchhos Reiki to be effective, one requires a sincere interest and background in certain Buddhist practices to achieve the desired results. Without this, the actual empowerments and ones practice will not be effective. As these teachings are translated and adapted, one can imagine that these teachings will, to a degree, evolve from the traditional model to a more accessible contemporary form.

MRS. TAKATA'S STORY

Until recently, a great deal of the historical teachings of the Universal Reiki system came from Mrs. Hawayo Takata. Mrs. Takata was a student of Chujiro Hayashi and is also believed to have known Dr. Usui, although she did not receive formal teaching from him. Mrs.

Takata, a Japanese woman, was the soul person responsible for bringing Reiki to the West in the early 1970s. As practitioners of Reiki, we owe a great deal to Mrs. Takata, for without her, the Universal Reiki system, as is recognized throughout the world today, may not have been.

Mrs. Takata had laid the foundation for Reiki in the western world, which in turn has benefited countless beings in their spiritual growth, healing and personal development. It seems that now humanity is ready to know more of Reiki, with its deep spiritual and esoteric tradition and how these teachings might further benefit humanity in our modern age.

When Mrs. Takata brought Reiki from Japan to the West, she took it upon herself to change the Reiki history to make Reiki more palatable to Americans. In retrospect, this was a very intelligent and cunning move. As you can imagine, in the conservative, highly Christian, post World War II America, a Japanese Buddhist energy healing system may not have been received too well. The traditional Reiki story has, in many ways, served its purpose and we are perhaps a little more enlightened with regard to foreign spiritual exports these days.

Here is one, (for there are many), of the traditional Western versions of Takata's story and how Reiki came to be.

Dr. Mikao Usui, a Christian minister in the late 19th Century, discovered Reiki. Dr. Usui was the Principal at Doshisha University, a small Christian University in Kyoto, Japan. One day he was speaking to his students of how great teachers, like Jesus, healed the sick. One of his students challenged him to show them living proof of these healing miracles reported in the Bible, and asked whether Dr. Usui had any ability to perform such feats of spiritual power. Dr. Usui, being an honourable man, confessed that he had no personal experience and that he could not teach his students these methods. He subsequently resigned his position to dedicate his life to rediscovering how Jesus healed. Usui believed that he would be able to study the best theology in a Christian country, so he travelled to America to study at the University of Chicago. Despite receiving a medical doctorate and studying theology, he still had not found what he was looking for.

Usui returned to Japan, determined to find his answers. He began visiting Buddhist monasteries, speaking with priests and scholars, but to no avail. Finally, he came across an Abbot at a Zen monastery who allowed him to study the secret writings of the Buddhist Sutras. It was within the Sutras that he found the formulas and symbols for healing, yet this was still not enough as he had no ability to activate this healing ability for himself. The kind Abbot advised him to meditate on the sacred mountain in the hope of receiving a vision. Usui trusted the Abbot and followed his advice. Usui made the pilgrimage to Mt. Kurama to fast and meditate for a period of 21 days. This he did, setting 21 stones in front of him to count the days. At dawn of each morning, he threw one stone away to mark the completion of each day. During this time he grew very weary from the lack of sleep and food, yet he remained vigilant in the hope of receiving his vision. It was not until the 21st day that he received the answers to his questions. Upon throwing the last stone that lay before him, he saw in the distance a strong beam of light travelling towards him at great speed. He grew very fearful at this display of spiritual power, yet he knew it must be the answer he was looking for. He remained very still and waited. This great light came and struck Usui in the forehead, overwhelming him until he soon lost consciousness. His spirit left his body and he was shown beautiful rainbow coloured bubbles of light, each containing the symbols he had seen in the Sutras. The lights entered his body and he was shown the mantras, the symbols and attunements for activating healing in others. Usui heard a voice say, 'Do not forget this, these are the keys to healing, do not allow them to be lost'. Some time later, he regained consciousness.

Usui was surprised to find that he no longer felt fatigued or tired. On the contrary, he felt euphoric and energized. Finally, after many years of searching, he had found the keys to healing power. He hurried down the mountain with great enthusiasm, looking forward to telling the Abbot of his experience. In his haste he tripped and fell, badly cutting his foot on a sharp rock nearby. Blood immediately began to flow from the wound. Usui placed his hands on the wound and great warmth flowed from his palms. Within minutes the bleeding had stopped, the pain had ceased and the wound had completely healed.

When Usui reached the bottom of the mountain he stopped at a food stall, as he had a considerable appetite from his fasting. Upon receiving his food he noticed the young girl serving him had been crying, and her face was red and swollen on one side. The girl told him between sobs that she had a very bad toothache, but her father could not afford dental treatment. Remembering how quickly his foot had healed, Usui offered to place his hands on her face. Again, great warmth flowed from his hands and in a few minutes the pain ceased and the swelling subsided. Usui then ate his huge meal with no trouble, considering his long fast. Later that day, Usui returned to the monastery and found the Abbot in bed suffering from a bad attack of arthritis. Usui held the old man's hands while he spoke of his experiences on the mountain, and within a short time all the pain from the arthritis had gone.

On the advice of the Abbot, Usui decided to work amongst Japan's poorest and most suffering. He returned to Kyoto and worked with the beggars in the slums. He worked there for several years, helping the sick and destitute. Although he had helped some of these people, many were returning to the streets in much the same condition as he had found them. Usui grew very disappointed and asked them why they had returned to a beggar's life. Their response was always the same, it was too much responsibility to work at a job and have a family. Returning to begging seemed an easier way of life.

Usui soon realized that it was not enough to heal a person's physical condition, that spiritual healing was vital in total transformation. Having ignored the beggars' spiritual needs he had denied them the appreciation for life and how to live in a new way. They had received this healing art freely and were not required to give anything in return, thus they simply did not appreciate the gift that was given. Usui then decided to leave the beggars and began teaching people who truly wanted to be healed. He developed five spiritual principles to assist his students in developing themselves in their healing:

- Just for today, do not anger
- Just for today, do not worry
- Honour your parents, teachers and elders
- Earn your living honestly
- Show gratitude to every living thing

As Usui travelled from town to town, he would carry a flaming torch during the day as a symbol of the light and spiritual teachings that he was offering. It became his calling card and his popularity soon spread. He acquired many disciples who would travel with him and assist him in his teachings. One of his principle students was Dr. Chujiro Hayashi. Usui continued teaching Reiki for the remainder of his life. Before his death Usui passed all his knowledge to his senior student Dr. Chujiro Hayashi so that Reiki could be passed onto others and not lost, as it had been in the past. Usui appointed Hayashi as the Grand Master of the Reiki lineage and Hayashi carried forth the work of his master in a similar manner.

WHAT ACTUALLY HAPPENED

The story just described is based on Mrs. Takata's oral tradition. Most Reiki teachers simply accepted Mrs. Takata's story as being factual until some practitioners began to research the origins of Reiki. In particular, I refer to Frank Petters' book, *Reiki Fire.*

In the original Reiki story, Mikao Usui is depicted as a Christian, teaching theology at the Doshisha Christian University in Japan. However, derived from Usui's personal notes, he was in fact a devout Shingon Buddhist. Further to this, Usui never taught at Doshisha University and was never a Principal of any school. Usui was also very sceptical of the Christian doctrine, although he later befriended a Christian physician, who became a mentor for Dr. Usui with his medical training. This is also described in subsequent chapters of Usui's manuscripts.

In Mrs Takata's story, Dr. Usui is also said to have travelled to the United States to receive his Doctorate in Medicine from the University of Chicago in the late 1880s. Other variations of the western story say that he was never a doctor and instead studied theology in the United States.

Recent research has determined that Dr. Mikao Usui never travelled out of Japan's sacred islands, except on two occasions, once to China where he studied Chinese Herbal Medicine and once to Hokkaido (Japan's northen island), where he had a short and somewhat arduous journey. This amusing story is later told by Dr. Usui in the following chapter. The Usui Memorial also states that Dr. Usui travelled extensively to some countries, though no mention of these journeys appear in his journals.

Indeed, if Dr. Usui had travelled to the United States and had studied medicine in the 1880s, the Medical Faculty of Chicago University had not yet been established. It wasn't until the 1890s that the Medical Faculty began in the city of Chicago. This was some ten years after Usui was meant to have studied there!

Usui was a Medical Physician and had received his

training from Western physicians in the 1880s, some of which were Christians who were sent to Japan with the first missionaries. The Chicago link, where perhaps Mrs. Takata introduced the theme, comes from one of Dr. Usui's friend, a Medical Doctor who he met in 1916. Usui's western friend had received his training from the then established Chicago Medical faculty.

Other aspects of Mrs. Takata's story describe Dr. Usui carrying a flaming torch when he visited villages, as a symbol of the 'light teachings' he was offering. This story however, describes the great Buddhist master Kobo Daishi who was responsible for founding Shingon Buddhism in Japan. The torch bearer, Kobo Daishi used this symbol as his calling card; he would carry a flaming torch during the day and was responsible for bringing Buddhism to Japan, not an easy undertaking. Kobo Daishi also brought with him the 'Tantra of the Lightning Flash', the essential teachings of what became known as Reiki.

Many variations of the western Reiki story also describe Dr. Usui's experience on Mt. Kurama. Some of these stories describe many sensational events, however, it is clear from Dr. Usui's manuscripts that certain insights and empowerments occurred during his meditation and retreat on Mt. Kurama.

Dr. Usui describes his time in retreat as being a time of contemplation and realisation. He also describes seeing certain images and receiving empowerments by the Reiki energy itself.

Usui writes... "These spheres manifested before me like bubbles rising on water and then I became aware of their importance and the methodology with which to employ them... (they) sank into me and bestowed upon me the power to impart this healing modality to everyone."

Dr. Usui visited the sacred mountain many times, to contemplate and regularly enjoyed visiting this sacred place. He also describes going to Mt. Kurama after his illness. It was here that he reviewed the turn of events which had occurred during his life, with his illness, his visionary experiences, the meeting of his Shingon teacher and the discovery of the ancient manuscripts.

These facts are being presented here, with the hope that existing Reiki teachers may gain a clearer understanding of the history of Reiki.

The new historical information that has recently come to light, with the discovery of Usui's original manuscripts, not only clarifies historical facts, but also sets a solid foundation to the origins of Reiki.

For all teachers and students who read this material, surely, it would seem unnecessary to propagate inaccurate information in light of this new knowledge. Perhaps with this new information, Reiki teachers around the globe will begin to embrace these new truths, which may in turn, assist in the establishment of a clear foundation and model practice of Reiki.

This information was derived from Usui's original manuscripts by the translators of the Dharma Society of the Glorious White Peacock and with the kind permission of Lama Yeshe Drugpa Trinley Odzer, the Spiritual Director of Menchhos Reiki International.

WESTERN UNIVERSAL REIKI

Although Mrs. Takata had received her final initiations from Dr. Hayashi in 1938, she did not prolifically teach Reiki until she travelled from Hawaii to America in the early 1970s. Once Mrs. Takata arrived in the United States, she began teaching Reiki to anyone she felt was sincere, and with the desire to extend this teaching to as many beings as possible.

Before Mrs. Takata made her transition in 1980, she had initiated some twenty two teachers in the third degree of the Reiki system. Mrs. Takata taught in a very different manner from one student to the next and, as a result, many of the original twenty two Western Reiki teachers have variations on their Reiki symbols, teaching methods and initiation procedures. These methods have been further distorted and fragmented over the last twenty years as the system has been disseminated throughout the western world. Most Reiki teachers in the western world today have their lineage traced to one of these twenty two teachers empowered to teach the Universal Reiki system.

"Prior to Mrs. Takata's death, a meeting of Takata's students was called. At this time, Mrs. Takata proclaimed Barbara Ray as her successor in the Universal Reiki System. Barbara Ray, studied with Mrs. Takata from 1978 to 1980, she later formed her own Reiki style which she called, 'The Radiance Technique'.

Mrs. Takata took it upon herself to teach Reiki according to her students' abilities and talents. She also tended to teach in an irregular fashion, and as a result, many variations in the Western Reiki System occurred. Today, as Reiki is passed to the next generation of Reiki teachers it becomes harder to encounter an intact Western Reiki System. This also accounts for the many and varied Reiki styles available today."

Since Mrs. Takata's death other teachers have assumed the title of 'Successor', which is also referred to as 'Grand Master'. Terms like 'Master', 'Successor', and 'Grand Master' have become new additions to the Reiki system since it made its transition from East to West. These terms were never used in Usui's day or as any part of the original Japanese Reiki system.

Below are the official twenty two students that Mrs. Takata initiated as teachers between 1970 and 1980.

Barbara Weber Ray
Phyllis Lei Furumoto
Beth Gray
George Araki
Barbara McCullough
Ursula Baylow
Fran Brown
Paul Mitchell
Iris Ishikuro (deceased)
Ethel Lombardi
Wanja Twan
Virginia Samdahl
Dorothy Baba (deceased)
Mary McFadyen
John Gray
Rick Bockner
Bethal Phaigh (deceased)

Harry Kuboi
Patricia Ewing
Shinobu Saito
Kay Yamashita
Barbara Brown

Lawrence Ellyard's 'Western Reiki' Lineage

Dr. Mikao Usui 1865-1926
Mr. Chujiro Hayashi 1879-1941
Mrs. Hawayo Takata 1900-1980
*Dr. Barbara Ray
*Gary Samer
Lawrence Ellyard

---

* Dr. Barbara Ray formed the Radiance Technique in the late 1980s as the authentic and original Reiki system as taught by Mrs. Takata.

* Gary Samer resigned from the Radiance Technique in 1990 and became an independent Reiki Master, and began teaching an independent Reiki style and system.

Chapter 2

'For I, Usui, am a river, I flow from the past to the future, through many turnings, yet I am that same river, in the past, in the present, in the future.'

— ***Mikao Usui***

EXCERPTS FROM DR. USUI'S MANUSCRIPTS

The following are a series of Usui's original manuscripts, letters and commentary on Reiki. These have been given with the kind permission of Lama Yeshe to further broaden the understanding of Reiki as it was taught in 19th Century Japan. Contained within the black lacquered box that came into the possession of Lama Yeshe, are countless documents and instructions of the original Reiki system. It includes the 'Tantra of the Lightning Flash', the spiritual methodology, Usui's practice of Reiki, countless techniques, practices and advice on healing, as well as personal anecdotes and stories of his daily experiences.

Much of the inner teachings of the system cannot be presented within this written format as they require initiation and a level of understanding that comes from training in Buddhist and Shingon traditions. However, the following is a letter that was attached to the 'Tantra of the Lightning Flash' that describes Usui's views of his day and some insight into how Usui came into the teaching of Reiki. It also conveys Usui as a man who clearly holds a depth of accomplishment with this practice.

(The following documents are transcripts of the original translations from Japanese to English as provided by Lama Yeshe, and their content has not been altered in any way, so as to preserve an accurate and authentic translation.)

DR. USUI'S LETTER OF ADVICE TO HIS SUCCESSOR, DR. WATANABE

This letter was written in 1925, just one year before Usui's death. Translated in 1994.

Usui writes :

I, Usui, have decided to set down in writing my motives and aspirations and the reasons why I have introduced this new spiritual science, which in reality is a very old spiritual science that had been lost and forgotten.

I was born the first son, the eldest of three brothers and two sisters to my father. My father was a lower level noble who, in his wisdom or perhaps cunning, had seen the handwriting on the wall concerning the old government of the military shogunate, which for the past fifty years before my birth had been toppling like a used and discarded table which finally came crashing to the floor, due to the wisdom and very well coordinated machinations of the Emperor Meiji, and his many supporters. This led to a change in the national attitude, which was striking.

From the time of the Naro period or even before, until the mid-19th century, Japan, although never admitting it, had looked toward China and in the western direction for its inspiration and culture. This was good, for the Chinese truly possessed it. Not only did they bless Japan with the basis of art, language, writing, the arts of calligraphy, and of course, the great gift of the Dharma, the teachings of Confucius, and the teachings of Lao Tsu, but they also imparted their penchant for the maintenance of stability and prevention of social change. This I feel, at least I felt at the time, was not good, as many young people did.

When I was sixteen years old I saw my first steam engine and was moved to tears at its symmetry, perfection, elegance, beauty and also function. Shortly thereafter there was an influx of Gaijin, western barbarians, into Japan. At first impression they resembled the demons of legions of old. With their light hair and reddish faces they looked to be the minions of the Lord of Death himself that had arisen from under the earth, and certainly the odour which emanated from them confirmed in most people's minds that they had not sailed from the East to Japan; these ocean barbarians, the round-eye, but had definitely sprung from the lowest realms of the Lord of Death.

However, I met a one, Mr. Philips, who was both a practitioner of his religion Christianity, an expounder of it, somewhat of a bonze, something known as a 'lay preacher'; and a medical doctor as well as a philosopher. As I became acquainted with him I found him to be a truly remarkable individual who, though totally outlandish in his behaviour and manners, nevertheless, I recognized as a fellow human being and one of great intelligence. I felt at this time, as many young people did, that I wished to learn all of this western knowledge, and would make any sacrifice, even sitting in the room with such a fragrant individual, to absorb his knowledge.

I found him curious of our ways and one day he asked the question that I had been waiting for. He asked, why were most people revolted by such foreigners. I joyfully gave him an answer: that they did not bathe. This startled and amused him and he informed me that he bathes at least once a month. I informed him that most Japanese, who were able, bathed at least once a day and that, unlike his folk, they suffered very little from carbuncles, boils and other skin eruptions. This amazed him and he wished to know how we stood immersion in such cold water each day, and did it not affect our health in other adverse ways. I am afraid that I broke into laughter and explained the concept that our baths were heated. He said that yes, he had taken a few baths that were heated by pouring a pot of hot water into a copper tub.

I told him that this was not the way that a civilized person bathed and invited him to enjoy my bath. He was terribly amazed and caused me no end of amusement when he entered the hot water and turned far redder than I had ever seen any individual before. In fact, his entire white body, which reminded me of the underside of an octopus' tentacle, when he emerged from the bath, was a most startling shade of crimson. However, he enjoyed the bath immensely and inquired if perhaps such a thing could be constructed for him. This was done, and it actually became a fashion among many of his friends, which was a relief to many of the students that were studying with them. In fact, I was congratulated by the student's family and presented with a rather large sum of money, at least for an eighteen year old boy, for having introduced the Gaijin to the proper civilized custom of bathing and thus establishing a great deal of 'Wa' in the community, which had formerly been upset by the remarkable and penetrating odours: these odours which seemed to be absorbed into any item they would come in contact with.

Mr. Phillips explained to me the doctrine of Christianity, which rather amazed me. It seemed to me to have very many similarities to the Pure Land of Amida. In fact, I was finally able to understand that perhaps Mr. Jesus had learned the doctrine of the Pure Land school and then had tried to explain it to his people, who were dull of wit and they punished him by crucifying him. The principle thing I could not accept of course, at that time or at any time in the future, was that man only lived once and had to obey a rather changeable, frivolous, unkind and vindictive God. As a Buddhist I knew that the Buddhas were all good, but during these years from the time I was sixteen until I was twenty seven, I rejected my faith and went after the great God knowledge; or at least scientific knowledge which had been brought to our country by the Gaijins.

I studied medicine and I also studied physics and I became a medical doctor through the kind teachings of

Mr. Phillips and other teachers, some from Princeton University, some from Harvard University, and some from the University of Chicago. I was granted a medical degree by decree of the Emperor and was allowed to practice with Dr. Phillips and his associate, a Dutch physician, Dr. Kerngold. I began to learn the finer points of surgery, having mastered pharmacology and the treatment and diagnosis of disease.

At that time, unfortunately, a cholera epidemic moved into Japan, which afflicted our people and particularly myself. I was stricken at the age of twenty-seven. The only treatment at that time for cholera was to let small pills of rolled opium melt under the tongue. This would slow the movement of the lower intestine and the individual would not dehydrate so much. The only other thing administered was a mild mixture of salt water and potassium chloride, mixed with fruit juice to prevent dehydration and expenditure of the electrolytes, thus badly affecting the sodium-potassium balance in the body.

Now I will say of opium that I found it at the time and later in my life, a way to open the consciousness in an artificial but effective way. I learned later that I could achieve all of this simply by meditation. However, at the time it opened my mind and I am sure that the illness also had this effect upon me.

One afternoon I had sunk into unconsciousness, at least was unable to move my body in any way, when I heard Dr. Phillips sadly tell two of his Japanese associates, Tome Dak, and I can't think of the other name, he was a nephew of Anoi Tetsuma; however, that I would not last out the night, that I was expiring and that my blood pressure was so low as to be negligible and that my heart beat was so weak that he did not expect my heart to last for the rest of the evening and into the night. This produced great sadness in the people there. It did not produce so much sadness in me.

I remembered my childhood teachings and thought of the Pure Land of Buddha Amida and that I would go there because I did have faith. In my mind I began to recite the Amida mantra 'Namo Amida Butso, Namo Amida Butso, Namo Amida Butso', and then I fell into a deeper semiconscious reverie and then into blackness; a dreamless state from which in the early evening I began to awake. I then noticed that I was not awakening in the hospital room, but in a place filled with light, the most beautiful of golden light. In my mind I thought to myself, 'I am dead and I am beholding the Assembly of the Pure Land.'

Well, on both accounts I was wrong. I beheld Mahavairochana. To his right was Amida. To his left was the Medicine King. Above the head of Mahavairochana was our first teacher Shakyamuni. They were surrounded by countless Buddhas and Bodhisattvas and their retinues. I immediately felt great sorrow for I remembered that I had rejected them.

Then Mahavairochana spoke to me and I beheld his face, the most kind and loving face, free from passion and attachment, yet filled with compassion for all sentient beings. He said to me, 'My poor child, you fear that because you have rejected your ancient and hereditary faith that we have rejected you. For a fully enlightened being, a Buddha, it is not possible for us to be angry or feel evil or ill thoughts at you. We only feel compassion for you and all beings who suffer in the churning ocean of samsara, facing the two terrors of birth and death.'

At this I was overcome with joy and happiness and at that moment I understood the commitment which these supreme spiritual beings have taken upon themselves for the well-being of mankind, knowing that each in the past had for many kalpas possessed a human body and had also undergone untold sufferings until they were able to put their heads above the water of samsara and step onto the dry land of Nirvana, reaching their Buddhahood, knowing all things, having experienced all things, and having developed that compassion which in any situation does not waver, but stretches onward until it is perfected in the supreme Buddha Mind.

As I observed the Buddhas and Bodhisattvas I felt terribly inadequate and humble before them. I prostrated many times and said to them, expressed to them my sorrow at having turned away from their spiritual science to the physical science that had been brought to us by the Europeans and Americans.

Buddha Mahavairochana smiled and said, 'But you have not turned away my child, for all learning and knowledge which relieves suffering is from the mind of the Buddhas.' At that I was again filled with joy and yet fearful that I had not earned my place in the Pure Land among the Assembly.

At that time Medicine King Buddha spoke to me and said I was a physician as he was, and that it would be my job, my mission, when I had recovered from my illness, to work to make a synthesis of both teachings. At that time, he expressed to me the old age teaching that the life energy, the Hari, is not separate from the body and that all physical suffering first emanates from the Hari and is due to karmic obscuration and past actions, which lead to the suffering. The surgeon's knife or the physician's pill can only temporarily relieve this suffering. For the individual to be truly healed, he must be healed of ignorance, hatred and greed. He must live a moral life, carefully walking the Middle Path and seeking enlightenment for his own self and others; that is the only true healing, that the Dharma itself is the only balm and medicine for the suffering of all living beings.

Then, when he had finished speaking, from his heart came the blue light of Probassa Vidurya, the lapis lazuli, and touched me. At that moment my mind and everything went blank and into darkness.

However, the next morning I awoke. To my physician's surprise and delight, no symptom other than the weakness of my illness remained. I quickly recovered. At that time it was unheard of for a person in my condition to have recovered so completely as to have no longer any symptoms of my ailment.

Unfortunately, I told Dr. Phillips and my colleagues of my dream. They gave it the explanation of the opium, which I was ingesting and the fever that I had and told me that a learned man of science could never believe such mythology and such things as were the provenance of the ignorant, unlettered peasant.

Later, about a week after I had recovered, I went to my bonze who told me quite a different story. On hearing the dream he became very angry and told me I was very arrogant; I was not a religious person. Why would I be telling such a lie about having such a vision and so on that not even the greatest abbot at the greatest temples had. How could I, a student, who was not even dressed in traditional Japanese manner, possibly have such a dream or experience? He called his guards; he struck me and literally threw me from the precincts of that temple.

Up to that time I had been raised as Tendai. However, almost immediately, I encountered a wonderful person who was the father of the person who became my best friend. He was Watanabe, the senior. He practiced a form of Buddhism known as Shingon. I took him as my mentor and explained the dream to him. Together we performed numerous fire offerings as a thanksgiving for the particular blessing I had been given to behold the faces of the Assembly of the Buddhas.

I began to meditate and study with Watanabe Bonze, and immediately my life changed. I became very calm. My desires and attachments began to break away and the obscuration, which I had held since childhood, began also to fall away like clouds before the morning sun. I continued to practice and received all of the lesser and some of the greater initiations of his Shingon sect. This was a great spiritual awakening for me and I understood that the dream within which I had encountered the Buddhas was only the beginning of the Path and was certainly not the end.

Keeping this in my heart I practiced as a physician and became rather well known in the area around

Osaka. Many people would come to me because they said I had within myself an ability to heal and that I had been born to this work. This is not uncommon among the peasantry who still have what many people refer to as superstitions; which I, just a few years before, thought were silly superstitions and now I believed were a perception and a wisdom that overcame the knowledge one learned, but a wisdom and understanding of the innate reality of things as they are, that goes beyond the normal perception.

When I was 34 years old I travelled to Kyoto and there in a bookstore I found an old lacquer casket, which had the chop of the Emorji Shingon Temple. Being a devout and fervent Shingon I felt it must contain some of the sutras or commentaries and I immediately purchased it for a small price. The outer casket was constructed of a very nice teak and interior of camphor wood. I took it home and discovered the treasure that I had found — one that I had been seeking without knowing that I had been seeking, and one that had been entrusted to me by the kindness and compassion of the Buddhas and the Bodhisattvas of the Three times.

It was at this time that I began to meditate on the material contained within the Tantra of the Lightning Flash. As I read and meditated, it became very clear to me that here was a spiritual system of healing that had been revealed from the lips and tongue of Shakyamuni Buddha, and that, through the ignorance and carelessness of man, had been lost for a time. It was my decision then that I would study and perfect this system of healing and perhaps in my old age pass it on to certain select students who would then promulgate it.

It became extremely clear in my mind at that time that this was the mission that the Buddhas had set me on at the time that I had the dream. This would be the path that I was to follow and this was the way that I, Usui, would gain the level of enlightenment, by promulgating and practicing this methodology that relieved not only the external, physical sufferings, but the internal sufferings and obscuration of humankind. This would go beyond both Chinese and European medicine. It was complementary and not contradictory to either system, but was the root of both systems for it had come from the Buddha's, and as all knowledge — both the knowledge of the Chinese and the knowledge of the Gui-lo, doesn't matter which — had also come from the mind of the Buddhas, particularly the healing knowledge from the Medicine King Buddha. So this I felt was what the dream I had experienced during my illness was concerning. Also this explained the miraculous recovery, which occurred when the physicians that were attending me had said that I would not last until morning and that I would not recover.

Those were the two events that changed the path of my life and led me to the fulfilment which I now feel as I set down this writing, so that my student Watanabe, the son of my mentor Watanabe, will be able to follow; and some advice I am giving him as well concerning conduct and concerning the way in which a physician, particularly a Buddhist physician, should comport himself in the relation of others, and in the relation also to his patients.

So I set down now so that he may have this in order to understand my feelings, why I have initiated the system which is to be called Rei Ki, and my feelings on the inner and outer teachings, and its application. I have given a little history about myself and I will give a little more probably as I go on, because what being does not like to talk about his past to others. It is a common human failing that is perhaps not a failing, but perhaps is a way to share experiences which we cherish with others; to share actually our life and life events with others, as a sharing, not a bestowal of knowledge as such, but a sharing on the common human conditions of life which all sentient beings that are at the human level experience. Perhaps from this commonality of experiences we can gain wisdom and understanding.

So here is some advice and things that I would like to say:

First, I want to discuss impermanence and change. I am not the same man that I was when I rose from my bed this morning, and when I rise from my bed the next morning, I will not be the same man. In fact, within my body, within a 24 hour period, my body is mostly water, and that water will be different water than I experienced when I rose this morning. This evening when I go to bed, most of that water will be different. In the morning when I arise, the water that was in my body yesterday will not be there, but the new water will be there which I have ingested by swallowing my tea, by eating my food and by drinking water itself, or the juices from plants and so on.

The proteins in my body will be different because many of them, the albumin will have passed through my urine and my defecation. Other proteins, which I have ingested from my noodles, from the wheat, from the fish

I eat, and from the meat that I eat — these are new proteins that I introduce into myself. My skin sheds many cells. Every time I move cells fall from my skin that are dry and are replaced by new cells. My muscle tissue is replaced, and so on.

There is a constant change in my body. There is constant change in everything around me. Now the practitioner of Reiki should be aware of this; should meditate on the impermanence of himself and should view death as inevitable. Not as a friend, nor as an enemy, but as an occurrence.

We have many occurrences in our lives. The friends that I have this year, some are the same and some are different than I had last year, and the year before, and ten years ago. Should I live another ten years, the friends I have will be different. They will not be the same people that I know now, because they too will have changed, and I will have gained new friends and lost old friends, either to simple separation or to death.

Many events occur. Impermanence is all about us. The sun rises and sets, the flower blossoms and withers, the grass grows and is cut back, the tree which has been growing for 300 years is felled by the woodsman's axe. All things are impermanent and subject to change. But you know, these things are only an illusion, a shadow. They are not a reality. They are only the reality, which we, through our beclouded minds, perceive. They are not the true reality that really exists around us; that true reality being the mind of all the Buddhas.

So death, being an occurrence, is also an impermanence. Yes, death too, is an illusion. Illness itself is a delusion caused by karmic obscuration. Perhaps even life itself is an illusion, caused by karmic obscuration. Think about that.

And think that I am also a river. I flow through time. I encounter the rocks and my banks, which cause my turnings. These are set before me by my karma. I flow yet around the rocks. Behind me is the mist from which I have flowed. Before me is the mist into which I flow. I am a river that flows through time. I have no beginning and I have no end and I am constantly in motion. Death is unimportant. Life is unimportant. Life itself is a link in a chain or ripple around the rock in the flow of my stream. For I, Usui, am a river. I flow from the past to the future, through many turnings, yet I am that same river, in the past, in the present, in the future.

Everyone is a river flowing from the past to the future. Every mind stream is unique, yet the same. The water, which flows in one river, is of the same substance as the water which flows in the other rivers. It is no different. Its formula is still H_2O. It might have different salts dissolved in it, and it might take a different course; it might be wide and lazy or narrow and urgent, yet it is still water. That is the unity of us all. The water in one river is the same as that in every other river.

If life is an illusion, how much more so is death an illusion? If happiness is an illusion, how much more so is suffering an illusion. These things have no real existence. They are phantoms, which pass through the mind. They are feathers blown in the wind. They are pebbles moving down a hillside. From the great emptiness all things have arisen and entered the great emptiness.

All things will return. From infinite light all things have arisen, and back to infinite light all things will return. The one permanent thing is the Mind of the Buddha, which permeates all existence.

And we are the Buddha. Truly it is only our own obscurations, our own clouded thoughts, our own non-understanding that separate us from total and complete enlightenment. The true practitioner of Rei Ki will realize this. When treating an illness he must realize the truth that illness is impermanent and is an illusion. It has arisen and it will pass. Perhaps death will occur, but that is an illusion too. And the illness will pass with death and the river's flow will continue. Onward and onward throughout time. One must view these things not as simply a segment or a slice. One must view things as continual and unbroken, the flow of the Mind stream throughout time. But then we must remember that time too is an illusion, and has no real meaning or effect on us.

These are profound truths and realizations that have come to me, and I know within me that they too are illusions and impermanent. I have experienced them. Perhaps others who will read my words will also experience them. But they too, have no permanence. This concept of impermanence must be fully impressed upon the mind of the practitioner of Rei Ki, the spiritual science. If it is not, then the practice is fruitless.

Before discussing the practice itself, I had wanted to say these things. They are the words of a silly old man and have no real meaning. But perhaps if they can provoke thought within you, my student Watanabe, then even though they are of little value, they will have served the purpose for which they were written.

I end this portion of the discourse now. I will continue it in the future. But remember that there is no past and there is no present and there is no future, for even time itself is an illusion and by a single clap of the hand, it too can be returned to the void, the one experience, the timeless reality which is the Mind of the Buddha.

Author's note: We see here from the man himself, the way Reiki came to be, its evolution from the Tantra and how Usui created the spiritual and healing way of Reiki.

The following article describes some of Dr. Usui's views on the various religions of his day and their interconnectedness.

FURTHER EXCERPTS FROM DR. USUI'S NOTES

I was asked by a friend, Ushima, why didn't I build a temple and why did I not begin conducting healing ceremonies. The answer is most simple, I am not a priest. I am a physician.

I believe the two can be combined in one person but my karma has not dictated that they combine in this humble person. I am 57 years old and even if I had time, I do not think I could absorb the amount of learning at my advanced age that it requires to become a bonze.

And my friend Watanabe bonze fulfils that function admirably since he studied since the age of 11 and even when he was a young man, made the walking pilgrimage through the country as a homeless brother.

Ushima has also brought up another important question that I had not even considered. And of course it is of serious importance. Ushima is Shinron. His primary devotion is Amida but for years he has also practiced our Medicine King (Medicine Buddha). We discussed whether it was necessary for him to give up his Shinron practice and begin to practice the Shingon form. Many of our people are Tendai still and their bonze and families object to their taking up Shingon when their religious history is that of Tendai.

Now I have given this much thought and since at the preliminary level of ordinary practice it does not matter, both Watanabe, Ushima and I feel we should discuss this. Watanabe is of the opinion that since Mahavairochana is not directly involved, that it is no matter from which school the practices are taken. Ushima on the other hand being an accountant by profession feels that standardization is of some importance. Neither Watanabe nor I feel this.

For instance, one of our best practitioners, who is from Panmunjom in Korea, Mr. Kim Yang Su, belongs to no Japanese school, but is a Korean Amidist of the tantric sort, the practice of his school being the one that has caused a certain amount of scandal lately in Tokyo and certainly has elicited disapproving glances from both the religious and civil authorities.

But I believe, and he has assured me, that their practices in actuality are in no way scandalous, nor are their doctrinal beliefs, but they are just misunderstood by the uninitiated and generally somewhat stupid populace, and even more stupid and rumour-mongering civilian authorities who for other reasons wish an excuse to dislike the Korean people.

Now his abilities at healing are extraordinary; his traditional Korean herbal medicine and Kundhyo massage techniques have produced results of a most extraordinary nature. Now that we are friends and a bond of mutual trust and respect has been established and is further developing between us, he has confided in me that since a young man he has used the energies of Medicine King even though without formal direction in his treatment agenda.

This has most heartened me and I believe that if this same energy of healing is exuded through him, having an origin in the training of the disciplines of his school, then perhaps most likely the origin of the Buddhist training and the methodology of manifestation and invocation is unimportant. My friend, Mariko Susuki, made a pertinent point when another matter of little importance was being discussed between her and her husband at their full moon poetry reading. That is, that there is only one Buddha Shakyamuni, no Zen Shakyamuni, no Shinron Shakyamuni, and thus so on.

So, thinking in this way, I must conclude, even though for most Japanese it might even be unthinkable that there is not necessarily a Shakyamuni for the Japanese, a Shakyamuni for the Koreans, a Shakyamuni for the Chinese, and even for the Europeans and Americans. After all, the Sutras do not tell us that he was born in Kyoto, but rather in some barbarous place in the Indian subcontinent. But of course, he must have been Japanese in a previous incarnation.

Following this line of thought, we must remember that Kobodaishi did not receive his teaching on Haihe

Mountain but in the barbarous realm of the pig and garlic eaters. But surprise! His teachers did not receive it in the Northern or Southern capital, but from adventurous, dedicated, devoted, kind travellers who, in order to work the benefit of the ignorant Han, had trekked long distances in adverse conditions from that barbarous place of mosquitoes, elephants and tigers, known as India.

I am sure many of our religious authorities, if not publicly, have probably privately, within the tightly closed closet of their own minds, questioned the wisdom of Shakyamuni to have been born in such disagreeable and barbarous place as India, when he could have just as easily been born in the only civilized domain in this world system: our beautiful civilized, sacred islands, inhabited of course, by the polite, unassuming, gentle, peace loving, humble descendents of the Sun Goddess.

After deeply contemplating these matters, I can only conclude that since there is only one Shakyamuni, there most probably is only one Amida, only one Fudo, and unfortunately only one Medicine King. Looking at the matter this way, and being well aware of the truth contained in the Sutras where the Sage states that 'the wheel is turned for every being according to their desires and mental structure' and that the validity of the Vehicle of the Elders is in no way compromised or superceded by the Great Vehicle. Nor is the Lotus Sutra, the foundation upon which Tendai is built, superseded by the Mahavairochana Tantra, nor as some of our Zen brothers would have us believe, superseded by the Heart Sutra; nor as our Honin brothers would have us believe, by the works of Honin, nor our Nicherin

Brothers by the repetition of the thought of a single mantra which I myself and many scholars have nowhere found in any of the Sutras or other teachings of Buddha, but apparently only was known to Nicherin.

Let us try then to look at the teachings with a broader view, using the simile that has always been used by the practitioners of the Bodhidharma that the Buddha, his teaching, and the Assembly are three precious jewels and each of these jewels has many facets. The facets of the Buddha for instance are Shakyamuni, Amida, Medicine King, Kannon, Fudo, Mahavairochana and Manjushi and so on. Each facet a Buddha radiating the brilliant light of his particular wisdom to benefit beings, and each facet of the Dharma jewel a different school, whether here in Japan, China, Korea, Siam, French Indo China, Ceylon, Tibet or India. And that the Sangha jewel is faceted. Each one of us is one of those facets, shining with its own light, working for the benefit of others and our own enlightenment.

Yet each of these jewels are not sundered or broken into pieces but remain a unity and that each and every facet is totally inseparable from all the other facets, for in order for their existence to remain they must be one.

In the light of this information, gained in meditation, I must only conclude that wherever the source or practice of Medicine King, Amida, or any other Buddha or Bodhisattva, it is valid and that the Buddha or Bodhisattva, disperses and makes available his energies through the individual practicing that system, irregardless of the country in which the system is promulgated and irregardless of the school which is promulgating it. So we may conclude that even Chinese and Koreans, the Indo-Chinese, and even those who follow the Way of the Elders can manifest healing energy from the Buddhas.

So let us set aside outdated sectarian views as we would discard a pair of old filthy and worn tabis and look to the essence of what we are practicing in place of the outward forms which our minds are so attached to, which we jealously guard as we would our family's history and upon which we place so much misguided importance.

DR. USUI, SPEAKING OF TIBET

We know that the Tibetans hold many secrets and have preserved portions of the Dharma that have been lost to the rest of the Buddhist world. Of course, this is because in their mountain land they were able to abide in peace and escape the wars and fightings that have so plagued both China and Japan. In this wondrous place of peace and contemplation, the Tibetan people have been enabled to put aside mundane matters and cultivate only the enlightened mind. That is why I am seeking to obtain Tibetan material, especially any material from the great medical college at Lhasa.

I believe that some of my missives may have reached the Grand Lama but I do not know this for certain. I am simply going to have to wait until my friend in India communicates with me again. I have certitude that secret texts exist which have not been promulgated in the rest of the world, and I am hoping to acquire some of these so that I may utilize their contents in my endeavours.

I would so love to travel to that place which most certainly must resemble Amida's Paradise of Great Bliss and drink from the incomprehensibly deep well of their wisdom in person, but age and infirmity prevents the realization of this desire at least in this lifetime.

So I must depend on my friends and co-searchers for truth who are utilizing the trade connections of the Indian merchants through Shigatse to Lhasa. So far, nothing has come out but I am sending to India now 100 gold British sovereigns and promising them to any merchant who can bring my friends valid medical texts written authentically in the old Sanskrit or even in Tibetan characters. Our circle here has decided among us that we will not accept texts in Chinese as they may be adaptations or perhaps non-authentic apocrypha, or even, considering the greedy propensities of certain individuals, outright forgeries.

So for the present time, we must remain patient and wait, hoping our prayers and expectations might be fulfilled by the infinite kindness and compassion of Medicine King, for I am sure our intention and aims are beneficial.

DR. USUI, ON DEATH AND DYING

Today an eight year old child died in my arms. It was struck down by one of those demonic conveyances known as the automobile. Its mother brought it to me and it died in my arms.

This led me to contemplate the matter of dying. As a physician I have seen the many faces of death and none of them caused me revulsion or terror, for it is the end of us all. A natural progression from birth through maturity.

In old times, the Samurai Lords proclaimed 'Let us pass as the cherry blossom falls in springtime.'

Now many wise philosophers have interpreted this that it means: Let us die in the blossom of youth before old age and sickness come upon us. I do not believe that this is what it means.

We would become bored if the cherry blossoms remained on the tree forever. It would no longer inspire us, nor fill our hearts with beauty and, furthermore, there would be no fruit. Rather, I believe, that in the springtime, first comes the bud, then the leaf, then the blossom. The blossom then fulfils its function and is fertilized by the happy bees. Its function then fulfilled, it passes, its petals fall to the ground and the fruit comes, containing within it the seed of new life.

This is the way that things have been and ought to be, for without renewal, there is stagnation. Then why do so many fear death?

The first is that they do not understand its true nature. The second and more important, if they are Buddhist or Christian, or perhaps Muslim or Hindu, they feel they have failed to live up to the moral precepts that their belief system demands of them. I will discuss this a little later.

The atheistic hedonist feels that he will be deprived of his enjoyment and simply go down into nothingness. I will deal with him first.

True, if one does go down into nothingness, one is deprived of one's pleasures. But one no longer suffers pain or heartbreak. I do not believe that nothingness is the end, but if I did, I would have no cause whatever to fear it.

I look back on my life to this point and see that the scant pleasures I have derived and experienced, are far outweighed by the suffering, struggles, pain and heartbreak that I have endured. Every day that I arise, I know that in some way I will experience pain. And I do not know if I will experience happiness or satisfaction.

Weeks go by without having the experience of something TRULY pleasurable. But not one day goes by without some sort of pain or distress. So why is life so terribly important? And why, if I believe, that all this would cease, should I have any fear of its cessation? Rather, it would seem that I would welcome it, so why should the atheistic hedonist fear death? The only reason I can think of is that the atheistic hedonist is not REALLY an atheist and perhaps there IS something waiting on the 'other side'!

Now let us progress on to the Shinto believer. I have never really met a Shinto who had any fear of death at all. The Shinto believer believes he or she simply becomes an ancestor or a Kami and no longer has to deal with the inconveniences of a body. One doesn't need a house; any tree or stone or even fence post will serve for the night. Some Kamis, who particularly like an area, will choose to abide there, with none of the inconveniences a human would have.

A Kami doesn't get wet with rain, suffers from heat or cold, or toil for his food. His religious descendants graciously supply it. If they fail in this duty for some reason, the Kami has ways and means of reminding them of their duty. Thus, the Shinto do not fear death.

As I was walking in the park near my home a few days ago, I heard two elderly lady adherents of Shinto discussing their coming transition. They were really looking forward to it.

They were considering all the juicy bits of gossip and talk they would be able to overhear in their non-corporeal form. Also, one of the ladies felt that her grandson-in-law could probably do with a good scare supplied by a thorough haunting. I find this attitude delightful and healthy and needless to say, most amusing.

Now, let's go to the Christians, those unfortunate souls. Whether Japanese or Western, the Christians believe that they only have one chance to make good, so to speak. To use one of their own expressions, if they do not walk the 'straight and narrow', then they will be damned forever.

From what I understand, the Islamic peoples hold approximately the same belief. What a terrible fate, because I am certain if this is really the case, the Christian Heaven is vacant of occupancy and its Hell is like an overflowing sake cup, dripping its contents from rim to table. Why do I say this?

Christianity is so filled with so many 'Thou shalt nots' and 'Thou shalts' that nobody would be able to fulfil the giri entailed therein. So, having stumbled on the 'straight and narrow' as any human being would, they are destined for eternal judgement and Hell.

Now, as a Buddhist, I must believe that the Christian God exists, but I believe that he is much kinder and much more compassionate than his proponents. I have read the New Testament and find that the image of Jesus portrayed therein is far from wrathful and vengeful. In fact, he spoke of love rather than condemnation, a lesson that many of his followers could well take to heart.

He seemed to me to be somewhat of a male form of our Kwannon, our Lady of Mercy, whose compassionate eyes gaze on all beings.

So, if one truly believes in this deity, Christ, then one should have no fear of death. Because it says that he will gather his elect to himself and to his father. Perhaps, however, it is fear of one's own shortcomings and willful violation of the ordinances that he should be obeying, that which lead to these fears.

I attended an Anglican Church service recently where the congregation fervently confessed that they had 'not done those things they ought to have done and they had done those things they ought not to have done'. My question was: Why? If they know what they are supposed to do, then they are surely capable of doing it and Heaven knows their deity has made it abundantly clear what they are not supposed to do, yet, apparently, as exhibited by their confession, they seem to have heedlessly done them anyway.

This is very confusing to me. What is even more confusing is that at the end of their confession, they solemnly promised not to do them again and to do those things they are supposed to do, then the very next Sunday, why do they say the same confession again? And the Sunday after that and so on.

Perhaps this is why the Christian people have a fear of death. My advice to them is to believe what their deity tells them, that he is forgiving, but my other advice is to try their best to do those things that he has told them to do and not to do those things that he has counselled them not to do.

After reading the New Testament, I think with some understanding, I feel that relying on the promises he has made and trying to do their best under the trying circumstances of this Samsaric world, they should have no fear about the future disposition of their Mind Streams.

Now to the Hindu. The Hindu, like the Buddhist, rationally believes that this life is only one in many. The Hindu is supplied with a list of do's and don'ts and sacrifices to make and rituals to perform. These are stated very clearly. If the Hindu is able to do this, then he has no fear of a good rebirth. From the Hindus I have met and communicated with, they don't particularly seem to fear death, because they strive to fulfil their religious deities very much as the Buddhist does.

Now we come to the Buddhist. The Buddhas have taught rules of conduct, which are most reasonable: to restrain from killing, lying, thieving, sexual misconduct, and the indiscriminate use of intoxicants, is most reasonable. The so-called Sixth Commandment, is even more reasonable: to try to better one's spiritual state while in the body.

I could give thousands of examples but I feel I don't need to, about the reasons that the first five should be obeyed. The sixth, any rational being can see the benefit and I don't think these are only for Buddhists. Virtually all of our Shinto believers have accepted and adopted them, admitting that the concept of moral conduct is truly important, as it is the basis for one's own progression along the spiritual path. Also, if the five are observed, one doesn't cause disharmony in the community and bring suffering upon oneself or others.

By simply observing these ordinances, the Buddhas tell us that one will gain a fortunate rebirth, so Buddhists have no true reason to fear death.

In summary, I believe that fear of death is fear of Self, and this should not be so. Truly, if one strives to live a proper life, as most people do, and give their best effort, then death should hold no fear, but be looked upon as a natural progression and renewal. For the Buddhist, it provides a chance to repair mistakes made in past lives and to move forward to greater realization. Thus, it is to be accepted and embraced as the normal order of human existence.

For those who fear death, I have this advice: We are told that both the Christian God and Buddha Amida are filled with compassion. How then, could they want even one soul to suffer? Therefore, it seems only correct to me and I do believe in their compassion, that they would not let one being suffer needlessly, nor would they desire to punish that being in any way whatever.

We are all joined together by the chain that is Life on this planet and to us, Life should be precious and a unity. At the same time, we should realize that death is an illusion and that in so-called life, we are a unity, so in death that unity is unaffected.

As a physician, I said that I had seen death, but I have also seen life and the multitude of stages between the two and I do perceive it as a Wheel whose hub is the grandeur of the universe.

When we were in the womb, we did not fear birth because, at that time, we had no comprehension of its meaning. It is the same now. Unless we have memories from previous lives, which few of us do, then we have no comprehension of the reality of death as a simple transformation. Since we did not fear birth, why should we fear death? It is just the doorway to rebirth. Doors have two sides and doorways lead from one room to another. Death is no more than a doorway and we should not fear to grasp its handle, slide it aside and pass through.

There is the story told in Buddhism about the peasant who pleased his Lord and inherited a great castle. The peasant had lived before that, in a one room hut. The peasant moved into the castle, but when the other Lords in the area came to visit him, they found him, his family and all his possessions living in the entry hall.

They asked him why and he answered that was what he and his family needed. To his amazement, they explained that there were many rooms filled with treasures and objects of beauty. Simply because he had not experienced them, that didn't mean that they did not exist, nor that they would hold terrors for him. They showed him the means to open the shoji screens and pass from one room to another. He was amazed and pleased and filled with joy at what he saw was his.

Of course, most of us are that man living in our single room, this life and not knowing the wonders, which await us in the other rooms of our castle. The kind Lords who visited him, of course, are the Buddhas, who explained to him that the castle had more than one room and, in their kindness, demonstrated to him the wealth of possessions that he possessed.

So let us look on death as nothing to fear, but an adventure, an exploration if you will, of a grand palace with many rooms. When the time for our transition approaches, let us not fear to grasp the door handle and slide it aside and pass through, experiencing the wonders of rebirth and spiritual evolution.

GUIDELINES FOR WESTERN REIKI MASTERS, WRITTEN BY DR. USUI

Usui writes:

The importance of Refuge in regards to the inner practice of Reiki:

The people in the West are inherently thirsting for a spiritual path. Christianity, except in a very few cases, has proven to be a dry spring from which they can only drink dust and debris. The introduction of the Inner System of Reiki, with its orientation in a superb quality of healing techniques and its deep and profound Buddhist connection, is that spring which many of them are unknowingly seeking.

The Buddhist refuge formulation and the active practice of Buddhist study and meditation must be accepted and agreed to before the student receives any of the Inner initiations. This Refuge and practice cover the ground of a dedicated, pure, and spiritual path, which requires of one a personal commitment for the benefit of all sentient beings in the six realms of existence. In order to successfully be a healer, and by implication practice the Inner System of Rei Ki, it is necessary that a person have this commitment. Each aspirant must without question sincerely take Mahayana refuge [the altruistic motivation to aid all sentient beings through the Buddha, the Dharma (spiritual methods) and the Sangha (the like-minded friends on the path)].

There is a very good reason for this based on simple logic, rather than superstition or any desire to 'recruit' people to Buddhism (which is forbidden in the Buddhist philosophy): The system of healing of the 'Tantra of the Lightning Flash' requires that the practitioner be able to partake of the stored psycho-magical energy that is stored within the 'Merit Storehouse' of all the Buddhas and Bodhisattvas. In order for the practitioner to partake of the psycho-magical, he/she must have taken with a clear understanding mind, refuge in the Three Precious Ones, the Buddha, the Dharma, and the Sangha, and must continue his or her learning of the Buddhist philosophy and practice. Furthermore, the practitioner must have awakened within him/herself the enlightened intention, (the intention to help others to health of mind, body and spirit, and the intention to gain enlightenment for the sake of self and others).

If this is not done, then there will be a blockage of the flow of energy from the Buddhas and Bodhisattvas, whether or not the person has received the initiation. Medicine Buddha himself (the Buddhist archetype of manifested healing qualities), in the practice of the lower levels of Reiki, freely gives of his energy at that level for the practitioner to accomplish the basic activity. But when reaching for the higher activities, seeking the energy necessary, not just to simply soothe and quiet an individual and work some benefit in that way, but actually to perform a healing and bestow the psycho-magical energy of the Merit Storehouse and make use of it, then we must have established a conduit for the flow of energy.

An example would be that at the lower level (the present so-called three degrees and mastership), it is like a kind Water Carrier who feels he can benefit a neighbourhood by taking water from a pure, crystal spring and bringing it to each home in a bucket. The spring is owned by a kind Daimyo (Lord or Master) who allows the individual to fill the bucket and then carry it to the people in the neighbourhood. That describes in simile how the lower level of Reiki functions. It is the teacher who has accomplished the Medicine King Buddha practice (Dr. Usui) who is the Water Carrier and it is the person who is practicing the three degrees of the Level One and his patient who are the recipients of this water.

However, once this first level is passed, it is the owner of the spring himself who has constructed a small canal from the source of the spring to his door. You can see the very meaningful and profound difference. The owner of the Spring of the Healing Water is Medicine Buddha. There are other springs as well: There is the Spring of the Cleansing Water, that is Mahavairochana. There is the Spring of the Water that gives better rebirth and also opens the way, washing away obscurations that prevent rebirth in the Pure Land, owned by Buddha

Amitabha. There is the Spring of the Water of Compassion of all of the Buddha's, whose owner, of course, is Kannon Bodhisattva. There is the Spring of the Water of Transcendent Wisdom and Knowledge, the owner of which is Manjushri Bodhisattva. There is the Spring of Deliverance from Rebirth in the Hell realms, or a spring that is preventative remedy for rebirth in the hell realms, but also the remedy that delivers beings who are in the Hell realms. That belongs to Ksitigharba Bodhisattva, Lord of the Sombre World. There is the Spring of Water that exercises the demons and the afflictions, the co-owners of that spring are Wei-To and Fudo Bodhisattvas. There is the Spring of the Water that repels the enemies, the owner of that is Hachiman Sama Bodhisattva, the great Suma Kami.

In order to utilize the waters from these springs in a meaningful, effective way, one must become a Buddhist so that one may partake of the Merit Storehouse. One cannot simply be Hinayana Buddhist because that is not a Merit Storehouse, that is the stair steps to selfishness. One must first take Refuge with knowledge and intent in a one-pointed manner, then one must confirm that refuge. The way that one confirms Refuge is to take the vow of the Bodhisattva. Then one is a Mahayana Buddhist. Then one may partake of the Merit Storehouse. This does not give you the Merit Storehouse, however, it gives you the ability to partake of the Merit Storehouse. Then, by bestowal of initiation into the deities of Reiki, you then have the Merit Storehouse. If you are not able to draw from the Merit Storehouse then the words, which you recite when you invoke the deities, are meaningless nonsense. They give honour to that Buddha when you praise him, but that connection, if you have not taken Refuge it is like a peasant sitting at home saying, 'The Emperor is good'. He is a far distance from the Emperor and perhaps the Emperor never hears these words.

After Refuge, when these words are said, it is as if a messenger carries these words to the Emperor saying, 'The Emperor is good'. But initiation is bringing you in the presence of the Emperor and you say those words to him and he is pleased by your homage and he therefore bestows blessings.

But in order to pass the gate of the Imperial Compound, as in the old days in Japan, you have to have permission that is written by an official of that court. That permission is the Refuge and Bodhisattva Vow. Then comes the official, your spiritual friend. You got by the gate, but there are all these vicious Samurai there who are guarding the Emperor. You are by the gate, but they say, "Do you have an appointment? Do you have an audience?" and you don't know. You say, "I love the Emperor and I came here." And they will say, "That's nice, but that is not enough. Where is your invitation?"

Then your spiritual friend comes and says, "The invitation is here to see the Emperor," and that is the initiation. Then you are conducted into the Imperial Presence, you praise him, say your panegyric, the Emperor is pleased and bestows his blessing on you.

It is the same with the Buddhas. Refuge makes it possible for you to approach the Emperor, but does not give you permission to do so. It simply creates the possibility. The initiation is what gives you the permission to approach the Emperor. But if you don't have permission to approach him, you cannot approach. And if you don't have the ability to approach him, you cannot approach. If you go to the gate and, even though inside waiting was an Imperial Official to conduct you into the presence of the Emperor, and yet you had no pass to get into the gate, you would still not go before the Emperor. The gatekeeper would say, "So sorry, I apologize, but you do not have a pass written out. I cannot let you in the gate to see your friend, even though the friend is waiting on the other side."

So that is an example of Refuge, the Bodhisattva Vow, and the empowerment. Believe me, it is not going to be an obstacle because for those people who are unwilling to make the commitment to take Refuge, the practice is not going to be successful even if they receive the initiations. There are many people thirsting for a spiritual path. The practice of Mahayana Buddhism, with its elevated concepts and universal compassion is that path they are looking for, although they do not know it yet. It is the path that will shelter, preserve, and instruct them, and at last bring them to enlightenment after empowering them to aid and benefit all sentient beings.

This teaching I am giving now can be revised as if it did not come from myself. It is just a teaching that can be given when students inquire about the importance of Refuge. But this teaching is particularly to understand the importance and the function of Refuge in regard to the practice of the Reiki system. This is very important. Keep it in mind and adhere to these concepts I have given you if you want the Tantra to be successful in the world.

CHARACTER OF THE PRACTITIONER OF THE INNER TEACHINGS OF REIKI

Usui continues...

The character of someone who is practicing the higher levels of the Lightning Flash should be one who is dedicated to healing. Not to self-aggrandisement, ego-satisfaction, or material profit. What is so amazing about this system is that all of these things will come to you: fame, fortune and recognition; if it is practiced with a pure mind and dedication to healing.

The individual who is initiated should be of good character, but most of all they should have the mental capacity to absorb the wisdom that is contained within each degree of the Reiki system. They should be stable individuals, not flitting from this healing system to that healing system. They should be willing to dedicate themselves to the perfection of one system before continuing on and seeking other systems.

The knowledge of healing that is contained within the Tantra of the Lightning Flash is vast and profound as the sky. It is as wide and deep as the ocean and it is inexhaustible. It is fine to use other adjuncts, such as massage, shiatsu and so on, to aid the individual. It is even proper to incorporate things such as Tai Chi, body movement and exercise, which when the tantra was written were unimportant because people had more physical activity in their day. This lack of physical activity does cause blockage in modern individuals, particularly the bureaucrat who has to sit in his chair for ten hours per day, or the executive who has to do exactly the same thing, using his mind and not his body. So these things are beneficial and can be incorporated. But other systems which indicate that they channel spiritual energy from this or that source of healing are unnecessary and a waste of time and endeavour, because within the system of the Lightning Flash all of this is contained.

If you own a warehouse that is filled with all manner of delightful possessions: fine foods, beautiful furniture and clothing and jewels, it is not necessary to go down to the fish market and acquire a new dead fish that is not as delectable, or as fresh, or as consumable as what you already have in your warehouse. In fact, it would be foolish, particularly since that fish might be old and tainted, or perhaps someone has intentionally put poison in the fish.

In your own storehouse you know the origin of every item, whether it is a food item, whether it is clothing, whether it is a cooking utensil, whether it is a map, whether it is a piece of furniture, or whether it is a garment. You know these have come from the highest manufacturer, the highest reputation manufacturer, and they are of the finest quality possible. Therefore, it is not necessary to seek from someone else's storehouse when you do not know the pedigree of the item that you are acquiring. This is not to say that you are to disparage the other merchant's merchandise. It is the simple truth that you have no need of the other merchant's merchandize because you yourself possess a higher quality, finer manufactured merchandize. So there is no reason to seek abroad for something which you possess already, which is of better quality than you can find elsewhere.

Also, if you are preparing a dish to serve to your friends, or for a party you are giving, you get the ingredients for the recipe. You find the squid, the octopus, the fish. You find the rice, the spices, the soy, the miso. When a good housewife is shopping, she knows the merchants that she is buying from. She has traded there in the past and she knows the quality of the commodity they are purveying.

Now let us say that this housewife has all the ingredients for her recipe to make a very fine thing for her friends and her husband's friends who are coming to dinner. Everything is there and sufficient to be cooked and go on the hibachi. There is a knock on her door. She opens and there is a peddler there. He says he has a wonderful ingredient that will improve anything she puts it with. She does not know the peddler. He may be good and what he says may be true, or he may be lying and what he says may not be true.

That prudent housewife is not going to buy his ingredient and combine it in her dish. Perhaps it could improve the dish, perhaps it could spoil the dish, perhaps it could poison those who partake of the dish. She is going to say, "No, I am sorry. I have my ingredients. I know where they came from. I don't know you, I don't know the ingredient. And besides all that, my dish does not call for your ingredient. I have all the ingredients, so I am sorry, but you must go somewhere else."

You are that housewife. The dish you are preparing is that dish that heals the suffering of all sentient beings, who are your guests that you are entertaining and presenting this dish to. So when you are preparing this dish, you must follow the recipe. You must be certain that your ingredients are known to you and know that the purveyor of those ingredients — all the Buddhas and Bodhisattvas — are of impeccable reputation, and the things which they purvey are of benefit and from an impeccable source. Then, when you prepare this dish that you will give your guests, all sentient beings, you know for a certainty that this dish will be tasty, nutritious, and will cause no harm, but only good.

The peddler who was at your door might be a good and beneficial person, and the ingredient he is selling might be a good and beneficial ingredient. But you do not know him. You do not know from where he came, and you do not know his intention in selling you the ingredient. But most of all, your recipe does not even call for that ingredient, so it would be stupid of you to buy that ingredient on his say-so, and put it into the dish that does not even call for that ingredient. No housewife on all the islands would do something like that in preparing an ordinary mundane meal for her family, husband or friends. So how much more important is it to not be stupid and incorporate some strange ingredient into your teaching when you already have all the ingredients and your recipe does not even call for this ingredient.

So that is what I wanted to say about that.

The other thing I wanted to say, about the people who will be practicing this path; they cannot be stupid housewives. They have to have an understanding that, contained within the system of the Lightning Flash is all that is necessary for the performance of the function. No strange new ingredients, perhaps brought by a Flying Saucer Person, perhaps brought by a self-important practitioner of some self-spring local belief, or anything like that should be incorporated into this system.

What should be incorporated into this system, if you feel a need to incorporate something, are those systems that have a lineage. Tai Chi, other physical exercises, means of beneficial massage, external allopathic medication such as the sulpha and the antibiotics in which a practitioner of that form of medicine would know how to administer in moderation for the particular problem the patient is suffering.

We must remember clearly and distinctly that all true healing medical knowledge springs from the heart of Burdurya Probassa Buddha, the Medicine King Buddha, and is not to be disparaged. But we must be sure before this is applied that it is truly a healing system and not something which has been created out of the fog and mist and floating gossamer of their own imagination. Allopathic medicine is a true system. Tai Chi is that. Shiatsu is that. Chiropractic is that. They are legitimate methodologies of healing. But there are many things that have been created out of mist and floating gossamer and falling feathers that are not that. So you must be careful to know which is that, and which is not that.

And this is what I wanted to say in this area.

In the other area, the individuals practicing must be stable individuals. What I mean to say very clearly without dissimulation is they cannot have their home constantly aroused, husband and wife fighting, or in the case of some people, wife and wife fighting or husband and husband fighting, or children fighting, or bills not being paid, and disruption in the household that unsettles the mind of the practitioner.

When one's mind is unsettled and worrying over other things; dwelling on interpersonal relationships, dwelling on the bill collector bringing the legal officials to the door, dwelling on the landlord throwing one out the door of one's dwelling, worrying about one's possessions being taken by creditors, worrying about one's wife having sex with someone else, worrying about one's husband having sex with someone else, worrying about having sex with someone else; all of these are distractions.

If one has these distractions, one is not able to practice the tantra with the proper clarity of mind and with full efficiency. So before practicing healing others, it is necessary to heal one's own life and to bring stability into one's life. So this must be kept in mind. If you see a student, no matter how sincere, that is having all of these problems, it is proper to give Refuge, but it is not proper to give initiation beyond first level. So the person's living must be stable. I am not saying that they must have money and a nice house and so on. They could be a mendicant, travelling the world for the benefit of beings. But they are doing that because they chose to, not because the landlord has put them out of the door or because the prefecture police are looking for them. They could be poor, they could be rich, they could be in the middle. They could be smart, they could be only a little smart; just so they are smart enough to comprehend the method and the methodology of the teaching. Whatever life they are in, they must have stability.

Rich people sometimes have less stability than poor people because these people are worrying about someone getting their money, and making more, and their mind is scattered with much worries about money; where poor people are not. But then, some poor people are wondering about where the next bowl of rice is coming from. That is not a good practitioner either. The rich person is not a good practitioner and the poor person must know where his next bowl of rice is coming from and not expect Reiki to provide it. The rich person must organize and put aside his business worries because all of these are distractions. So that is all I am going to say about this. That is all I have to say today. Saran ara. And this time I mean it.

USUI'S STORIES OF HEALING LOCALS OF NEGATIVE ENERGIES

(Author's note: The following stories describe how negative experiences can greatly impact on locals. Various solutions to these examples are explained in the second section of this book in Chapter 10 on Clearing Rooms and Bringing Reiki into a room. These following examples illustrate how negative energies, although not present in their origin, can nonetheless, affect individuals within their domain.)

Usui writes:

As Buddhists, we know that irrefutably spiritual vibrations

of either a negative or positive source can most certainly and irrefutably affect both the spiritual and physical well-being of an individual.

The first disruption, of course, originates with one's own negative karma. Since it is a primary cause of illness and the root basis for suffering, I do not include it in my enumerations, but will examine external spiritual causes of vibratory or subtle disruptions.

'Though long past and forgotten, the piteous sighs of the dying warrior on this blood-soaked ground, yet but standing here causes an unearthly chill to arise in my blood.'

So spoke a Chinese poet of the Sung Dynasty. He was travelling through China and stood upon a famous battlefield where an ancient battle had been fought. Such death, carnage, and suffering had taken place there that obviously the very rocks, earth, trees were imprinted with extremely strong negative vibrations, so that hundreds of years later the poet's mind stream was negatively affected by the incidents that had occurred.

When I was young and living at home there was a house of the 'Y' family. Around 200 years ago a murder had taken place in that house in one of the rear rooms. A Samurai returning from his service to the Emperor had come upon what he thought was his wife and her lover. In his frenzy of wrath he had pulled his sword and beheaded both. His wife then entered and he discovered to his horror that he had dispatched, not his wife and her lover, but his wife's beloved sister and his brother-in-law. Doing the only honourable thing he committed sepukko (suicide).

After that no one had been able to live or sleep in that room. Anyone spending any time in that room would be overcome with an all-pervading sense of dread, horror, and terror, whether or not they were aware of the unfortunate events that had taken place in that room.

Numerous attempts were made to use the room for food storage, but none were successful. The food would quickly spoil or was infested with insects or rodents.

It wasn't until later when I was much older and I discovered the efficacy of the purification ceremony that I was able to purify that room and set it aright, and restore its harmony.

Now I would like to mention that the room had no ghosts. It had been purified and exorcised by numerous Buddhist and Shinto ceremonies over the years. What had occurred was that the negative vibrations of the unfortunate tragedy that had occurred there were imprinted on the very timbers and stones, and influenced anything occurring in that unfortunate room. Those people who were able to fall asleep had dreams of flashing swords, blood, and rolling heads, and the woman (the Samurai's wife) screaming in terror and expressing her horror at what had there occurred.

Another house in our neighbourhood belonged to the 'S' family. About 150 years ago young Lord 'S' had taken to wife Lady 'M' and they lived in conjugal bliss. After a while Lord S's father died and Lord S's mother came from the country estate to live in town and brought with her one of her ladies-in-waiting, Lady 'K'. Lord S's mother did not care for Lady M and convinced Lord S to take a second wife, in particular Lady K. Disharmony immediately reigned, so much so that Lord S contrived protracted visits away from home on various business.

One such trip ended in Lord S's death away from home.

Yet disharmony still reigned, even after Lord S's mother's, Lady M's, and Lady K's deaths. Disharmony still reigned among Lord S's two sons and five daughters and continued to do so until quite recently when I performed a ceremony with the purifying and pacifying water, which I will teach to you at a later date. As what I am trying to impress upon you is not necessarily the efficacy of the ceremony, but that various locales and dwellings can be infused with negative energies.

I will relate another story. Approximately 300 years ago a local Lord raised very fine war horses. These horses he housed in an elaborate barn and ordered the greatest of care which he oversaw himself. One day one of his Samurai grooms through negligence allowed one of his prize stallions to break its leg and the horse was subsequently put down. The Samurai groom was whipped off the Lord's property and planned vengeance in his heart.

One night he and some Ronin cronies of his entered the barn, slew two grooms and all of the horses. When the Daimyo awoke the next morning he visited the barn and saw the carnage. He knew the cause and afterward hunted down the malefactor and his accomplices and quickly dispatched them before the court of Lord Yama.

After that even though all blood had been thoroughly cleansed from the building and the building exorcised by both Buddhist and Shinto ritual, no horses would prosper there. They would become exceedingly nervous, high strung, and even the most sedate on spending time in that building would become vicious and attack grooms and their attendants. The building fell into disuse for some years and another stable and barn was built by the Daimyo without any similar problems or disasters occurring.

About 75 years later the barn was refurbished and turned over to a sword maker. Shortly thereafter, one night while working late the Master went insane, slew his journeyman and apprentices with the sword he had just made, and took his own life.

The ill-fated building again fell into disuse for about 50 years when one night a band of soldiers of the Shogun, returning from the provinces to Yedo (Tokyo) after a successful mission to the provinces on behalf of their Lord, sheltered in it from unseasonable weather. As all soldiers will do they drank some saki and engaged in gambling. A dispute arose and eleven of the soldiers were slain by their comrades. This of course led to the local Daimyo holding a court on behalf of the Shogun and ordering the remainder of the troop executed.

The building then again fell into disuse. About 25 years later, also in the midst of a storm, three Shingon, two Tendai, and one Zen monk took shelter in the building. They all were collecting donations and travelling about on behalf of their respective temples. The one surviving Shingon monk told his story of the unfortunate event that had occurred.

They all were well supplied with provisions, the Tendai monk with a bit of saki. They built a cosy fire and had a rather sumptuous supper of rice, fish, and vegetables, and a moderate amount of saki. They then about 11 p.m., after prayers to the Lord Buddha, fell asleep. Apparently the Zen monk woke during the night and decided to acquire the other monk's treasuries for his monastery. Disregarding all the teachings of Lord Buddha he took his small but sharp eating knife and slit the throats of the brother monks with the exception of the one Shingon who, having been a former Samurai, overpowered the craven assassin, rendered him unconscious, tightly bound him, and delivered him the next morning to the Daimyo, who then ordered a trial and investigation into the awful occurrence.

The Shogun and religious authorities dispatched officials from Yedo immediately, one of these being my friend Watanabe Bonze's grandfather. A thorough investigation occurred, also a very unnerving incident: while examining the building an altercation developed between the Tendai Abbott, a saintly man of 87 years known for his piety and holiness, and the very kind and gentle Imperial Official. The elderly Abbott managed to knock the Imperial Official down and would have dispatched him with a rock, had the others not intervened.

All quickly exited the ill-fated building, and when the elderly and saintly man had recovered himself, like the poor Zen monk, could not explain what had come over him. Fortunately historical records had been kept of the horrible occurrences in the building and it was decided by all that the building was contaminated beyond redemption and the poor Zen monk was not responsible for the heinous actions he was caused to commit under the baleful influence of the ill-fated building. After tea and a very short discussion, the building was condemned to death by burning as a causative factor.

The stones of its foundation were scattered and its ashes collected and thrown into a nearby river.

Now two years ago in the company of Watanabe and his son after hearing the story, I visited the spot. The vegetation in the area had an unhealthy look and was inhabited by many varieties of noxious stinging and biting insects. We were even attacked by a number of wasps and had to hurriedly leave the area.

The next day armed with the Water of Purification, I cleansed the area. Last month I again visited the spot. The noxious insects were gone and not only had the vegetation returned to normal, but was luxuriant and fragrant.

Obviously this unfortunate locale had been ill-affected by the acts of the vengeful groom which had led to the unfortunate madness of the sword-maker, which reinforced the baleful influence, which then led to the violence and viciousness of the usually well-disciplined troops of the Shogun, whose vicious acts even led to more reinforcement of the baleful influence, which led to the murder of the monks, and the saintly Abbot attacking his close friend, a cousin of the Emperor, who himself, though a refined and gentle young man also became contentious and violent while under the influence of this terrible place.

It was very clear to me and everyone concerned later that this place was so infused with negative vibrations that it could obviously transmit and give rise to negative actions by its own ablative of contagion.

Now all of us have visited Kamakura and I have never met anyone, even a foreign barbarian of the Christian religion, who did not feel a sense of peace and goodness. Just as a place can be infused with negative energies and vibrations, so obviously it can also be infused with the positive. We have examined how human actions of violence and discord can cause disharmony, violence and murder to occur. At the same time positive actions and the beneficial actions of the Buddhas and Bodhisattvas and their infinite compassion can cause an area to be infused with positive energies. I have found that Reiki can be used to influence an area or a habitation with these positive energies, particularly the healing and compassionate energies of Medicine King Buddha.

THE TRIP TO HOKKAIDO

Excerpts from Dr. Usui's manuscripts

Today I returned from my trip to Hokkaido and am suffering from complete exhaustion in body, mind, and spirit. It began with a train ride to our port of embarkation that I truly enjoyed. We then spent the night in Tokyo itself at a small hotel.

The reason for this trip was only to please Watanabe Bonze; his mother's brother owns a small hunting lodge on our Northernmost Island. Hunting has never been a really Japanese pastime as far as I am concerned, and most certainly has not been an avocation of mine, but to please my friend and his son, I chose to give in to their entreaties and spend one week in their and their relatives' company.

Personally, I consider it a most brutal thing to hunt and murder wild creatures in their natural environment. I feel it is much better to simply observe them, as they occupy their niche in the magnificent panorama of nature. To end their lives in such a brutal manner in such a peaceful and lovely setting is murder to my sensibilities. But to continue: we finally reached our port of embarkation that was terribly dismal. An early fall fog had engulfed the entire Northern portion of Honshu, so we set sail, or perhaps I should say set steam, into what seemed endless gray mist. The crossing, however, was smooth and we arrived on Hokkaido in the early evening.

Our host, who had not appreciated our large amount of baggage, had provided two open carriages. This necessitated the hiring of a small wagon from one of the local draymen. After considerable confusion and a certain amount of impatience, though politely masked, on the part of our hosts, we were away to the country lodge.

Unfortunately our host had not anticipated the inclement weather and for an hour and a half we suffered drizzle. One of the open carriages did have an extendible cover; as the drizzle increased to our host's insistence that it would not, an attempt was made to raise the cover.

This resulted in all of us being showered with dust, twigs, and a number of years' collection of leaves. As success seemed imminent, a large tearing sound was heard and the top split; however, it did afford a modicum of protection. If one leaned far enough back, or for the passenger far enough forward, one escaped the worst of the rain, to which the drizzle had turned while we were delaying to try and raise the cover.

As we neared our destination a constable on his horse met us. He had been sent by our host's wife and mother to ascertain if some mishap had occurred on our journey, as we were now two hours late. We assured him that other than being soaked to the skin and chilled, we were fine.

On arrival at our host's home, we discovered his wife, mother, maids and daughter, though exceedingly polite were more than displeased at our late arrival. An elaborate meal of local delicacies had been prepared, and had been awaiting us. Since much of it consisted of fresh sashimi, much of it had been spoiled. We satisfied ourselves with the dry somewhat inedible remains and I was most happy to acquaint myself with my futon.

The next morning dawned ominously gray. Horses were brought after a hasty breakfast of cold rice. We mounted and rode into a gloomy forest, seeking to find some innocent creatures to murder. After four hours of riding and walking in rain, drizzle or fog, it seemed that the wild creatures were much more intelligent than we, for in all of that time, we had seen three birds who looked as bedraggled and dejected as we. It was then discovered to our host's horror, that the hibachi, the charcoal, and tea ingredients had been somehow left behind, but we had cups and plates and bowls.

We then trudged another three hours home without refreshment. When we arrived at our host's, we found that we had not been expected for another three hours, so no food had been prepared. Our hostess, though smiling, was furious. We could all sense this, particularly her husband who walked and spoke very softly. A quick dish of noodles made of miso and tofu was prepared with promises of better things to come. I quickly, after eating, retired to my room and prepared myself a salt-water mild carbolic gargle, as my throat was getting sore and not surprisingly, I was beginning to develop a cough.

A storm of terrifying proportions then commenced at about 8 o'clock that night. I had dozed fitfully off with a slight fever when my window blew open and I woke to discover that an icy trickle of water had been falling on my hips and legs from a leak in the ceiling. Fortunately two comforters had been provided and I had not made use of one. I carefully moved my futon to the other side of the room, drying myself and making use of the second comforter which, having remained unused in its cupboard, was as dry as could be expected in such a miserable climate.

About an hour later, I was roused by my host and told that a dinner had been prepared. The storm was raging outside. I felt I did not want to leave my futon, but politeness forced me to rise and dress, refresh myself and then enter the main room for dinner.

Knowing that I had been entertained by Westerners, my hostess had attempted, and I do say attempted with dismal failure, to prepare a surprise Western meal. This consisted of potatoes which I never really had become fond of, boiled to an unrecognizable mush, beet root pickled in sweetened rice vinegar, and a piece of venison fried in one solid piece and the consistency of a piece of old untanned dried leather.

Of course, I had to eat this, for courtesy forbade me to leave the table in disgust. Sake was served and although I usually only partake of one small cup, I decided for the sake of my health and hoping that perhaps my fever would be forestalled, I partook of a number of servings, and I will say that my mood considerably improved.

We spoke of the war raging between Russia and Japan, and how foolish the Russians were to think they could possess any of the territory of the Sacred Islands.

At about one in the morning, I repaired to my room looking forward to a good night's sleep when I discovered that the small leak had developed in my absence to a veritable torrent, thoroughly soaking the floor and the futon, having overflowed the chamber pot I had placed under it. Furthermore, three more leaks had developed, making the room uninhabitable.

I returned to the main room of the house and informed my host of the problem. As nothing could be done during the raging storm, my hostess's youngest maid was evicted from her room to sleep with my host's youngest daughter and I was given her room, which was snug and warm, but due to her devotion to one of the local Kamis smelled so strongly of the cheapest incense to which I am terribly allergic, that numerous times during the remainder of the night I feared suffocation.

My host's servant, who informed me that the storm was over and a delightful trip to the nearby village had been planned, awakened me quite early. I might add here that during the night, the combination of the overly-sweet odor of the incense, the sake, and beet root, not to mention the leather-like deer flesh, had begun to wage war in my stomach and I had to rush outside during the worst part of the storm to expel at least one of the combatants from my body.

I returned and was able to finally warm myself and return to sleep for what seemed a moment or two, before the cheerful man-servant wakened me and informed me of the further torture my host had planned for me.

After a breakfast of sweetened gruel, which did my stomach a considerable amount of good, we boarded the open carriages again in a light mist and rolled through the mud to the country village. There, some of the local handicraft of some of the aboriginal peoples could be purchased, and to my delight I found a lovely tea pot with cups made by a local potter and purchased it as a gift for my mother. To my complete joy I was able to purchase a woolen kimono, padded with further layers of wool and lined in silk. I considered the purchase of this item the pinnacle of my holiday.

After a substantial lunch at the local inn, which I thoroughly enjoyed, I began to believe that I might derive some pleasure from my visit to Hokkaido. How terribly mistaken I was.

Half-way from the village to my host's home, was a small Shinto shrine to the same local goddess that the maid so fervently worshipped. Nothing would do unless we stopped. I should mention at this point that the sky was beginning to take on an ominous hue, which to me presaged more unfortunate weather.

My host, claiming constant habitation on the island since birth, assured me that we had plenty of time for a visit. We arrived, made obeisance and gave a small donation, whereupon the priest in charge of the shrine produced his blind and deformed daughter, who he claimed was a famous medium in these parts for the Kami who inhabited the shrine, and who had a message for all of us from 'the other side'.

For a moment I will digress here to say that I believe that there are those who have been blessed both by the Buddhas and the Kamis with the ability to communicate with the spirit world. Of this, I have no doubts whatsoever. However, there are those, and one finds them generally in poor rural shrines, who boast that they have the ability and do not. One only feels pity and sadness for them, considering the karma they may generate by giving false messages from one's ancestors or purported local Kami.

But to return to my sad and tragic narrative. The father then began to chant before we could make our exit and the daughter began to mumble and twitch. The assistant priest than appeared with paper, ink, and brush and began to interpret the message.

I was told to my horror that I would travel extensively to America, Europe, and China. This truly filled my heart with terror considering that this excursion, only a short one, was fraught with so much suffering and inconvenience. I resolved at that time that should Lord Mahavairochana grant me a safe return home, I would never travel any distance again.

Fortunately, I did reach home safely and upon arriving had a Saito Goma performed in thanksgiving for my safe return, and then strengthened my resolve into a vow that I would never travel extensively again.

But to return to my narrative: For approximately three hours the poor child twitched and mumbled, as my host's wife's mother had a great deal to communicate from 'the other side'. And my host's great grandfather had a similarly lengthy communique for my host. Finally the poor child fell into a swoon and was carried away by her mother and sister. We made a further donation and returned to the carriages.

We had not travelled half a mile before the sky veritably opened, drenching us with the heaviest rain yet. Within approximately half a mile of our host's home, one of the axles of the carriage in which I was riding fractured, the wheel came loose, and I was dumped from my seat face down in the mud. My host and his servants were able to un-stick me, clean me a small bit, and place me in the other carriage, promising me a hot bath as soon as we returned home.

Upon our arrival I was sadly informed that the wood used for the bath had become so soaked in the rain that it would not ignite. Some water was heated on the brazier and I washed as best I could, looking forward to wrapping in my new quilted kimono, only to discover that it had been left in the disabled carriage. A servant was sent for it and it arrived anon somewhat damp. It was then dried over a brazier for me and I wrapped in it feeling slightly revived by the dinner my hostess and her servants had hastily prepared.

I then discovered that during the small break in the weather, the roof of my room had been repaired and fresh futons and quilts had been provided. I, then pleading fatigue, returned to my room and slept very well.

The next morning I woke quite ill. The repeated soakings with cold rain had their expected effect. I rubbed my body thoroughly with camphor ointment, and taking from my pack the proper herbs with which I had providentially provided myself, gave the servant instructions on preparing me a tea.

I also dosed myself with syrup of ammonium chloride and ingested a small quantity of methyl morphine for my cough. I remained in bed for two days and having somewhat recovered was informed that we would hunt in the afternoon. A very wan sun looking as insipid as I felt had broken through the clouds and did provide some warmth.

After a small lunch we set out at about 1 p.m. and within 15 minutes had taken three pheasants. It sickened my heart to see such beautiful birds shot from the air to land in a broken heap on the moldy ground. But this was not the only horror in store for me.

In about an hour we came upon a grazing doe that was immediately dispatched by my host. It was only then that we noticed the two fawns that had been born the previous spring. Having felt the venture successful, we returned and one of the pheasants was prepared for our evening meal.

Claiming a return of my illness, I excused myself from partaking and satisfied myself with some fish broth and noodles. I do not feel that I possibly could have partaken of the pheasant whose brutal and untimely death I had witnessed that afternoon.

The next day I remained in bed, so I did not have to participate in a second expedition, again claiming that my illness had returned.

More pheasant were executed that day as well as a small fox whose winter coat was coveted by my hostess for a Western style wrap. It completed the set of five necessary for the construction of the garment. The next day we were scheduled to leave and in the morning were conveyed without further incident to the ship where we embarked for our return home.

We had travelled only a short distance when a storm blew through the Strait causing our craft to move simultaneously in all directions at once. I became exceedingly ill and remained so for the rest of the voyage. Upon arriving at the shore of blessed Honshu, I was unable to travel any further and took refuge in a local hotel, built in the Western style with a roof that didn't leak and a large white porcelain tub in which I immersed myself for approximately three hours.

The next morning I awoke terribly ill and had to remain three more days for fear of my health deteriorating. Watanabe Bonze remained with me while his family returned home.

Feeling a little better on the fourth day, I visited my friend the British doctor, Dr. Winston Caine, and his brother John, a non-conformist missionary. The good Dr. Caine then dosed me with a concoction of calomel and other unknown ingredients.

When I returned to my hotel I discovered that my return home had been delayed two more days by the effect of the medication. Finally, reaching my own dwelling, weak and exhausted and still suffering from 'le gripe' (a cold) and perhaps incipient pneumonia, I retired immediately to my futon and the care of my own servants.

As soon as I had sufficiently recovered, I had a Goma performed in thanksgiving and seriously vowed never to travel extensively again.

THE VISIT OF THE TSAREVITCH

Excerpts from Dr. Usui's manuscripts

In the ill-fated and inauspicious summer of 1890, I travelled with my friend Watanabe and my father for a visit to the shores of Lake Biwa and the town of Otsu. Six months before, my father had secured rooms at an historic Inn, not knowing that during the ensuing summer, there would be a visit by the Russian Tsarevitch Nicholas. Looking back on those events, I am wondering if they perhaps presaged the unfortunate conflict with Russia in 1904 and 1905, after Nicholas had ascended the throne of all of Russia.

The first thing that occurred was that the manager of the Inn tried to repurchase our reservations, but to his dismay, even though he offered twice their value, we were adamant on staying our ten days. Otsu was extremely crowded due to Nicholas' presence. The town was filled with enough police to fight a small war, both secret and public.

There were numerous gaping Westerners from all over the country, as well as that class of Japanese who will travel far to see a tailed frog or a two-headed bovine. The attraction of a foreign dignitary has never moved me. But to some people whose lives must be so boring as to be almost intolerable, anything will be a reason for travel simply to break the monotony of their lives.

We found it disagreeable and inconvenient as the prices in most shops had tripled or quadrupled during the Russians' visit. Also various parts of town and even the lakeshore itself were quarantined whenever the Russians were present.

All the criminals, drifters and con men had been rounded up and expelled before our arrival and much care was taken to improve the already beautiful aspect of Otsu. Over my protests on the day of the Imperial procession I accompanied my father and Watanabe to a street corner to view the Russians. It was fortunate that I did. The procession was led by troops of our own Imperial guard followed by the very large Russians in full dress uniform and their band. This was followed by another group of Russians wearing blue, who were apparently their Imperial guard, then carriages containing our Imperial officials and local notables, and then the carriage of the Russians.

When the carriage was approximately forty yards from me, one of the police left his station and with a sword struck at the Crown Prince's head. The unfortunate and deluded man was named Tsuda Sanzo. One of the rickshaw pullers saw the blow coming and was able to somewhat deflect it. Two of the Russians jumped from the carriage and began to struggle with the assassin. Two other rickshaw pullers grabbed the assassin's legs and the group wrestled him to the ground.

The Crown Prince's plumed military headgear had been knocked aside and blood was pouring down his face from a cut on his scalp. My instincts immediately took over and I rushed toward the stricken noble. A number of police immediately restrained me but my continued shouting that I was a doctor calmed their fears that I was perhaps another assailant and they allowed me through. I noticed that he was barely conscious and had an extremely elevated pulse and respiratory rate. He was carried by his own guard into the lobby of a nearby hotel and I was hustled along.

A room was immediately provided and the Tsarevitch was taken there. I accompanied him, followed by a number of Imperial officials, as well as the police with their revolvers drawn. He was placed upon the bed. I was then able to loosen his jacket and give him a thorough examination.

The cut though shallow, was bleeding profusely, and I tore hasty bandages from a sheet provided me by the management and cleaned the wound. My father had rushed back to our Inn and delivered my medicine bag about ten minutes later. I was quite fearful for the foreigner's life, as his pupils were unequal and he was perspiring profusely, though still only semi-conscious.

I feared that a subdural hematoma might be forming, as the blow had been struck on his left side and he was experiencing small tremors and spasms in his arm and the leg on the right. I am not a head surgeon, but I feared that surgery might be necessary to relieve the pressure, however, at that moment I called upon Medicine King Buddha and was told what to do. I placed both hands on the left side of his head and spread my perception inside of the injury. I noticed the formation of a small hemotoma, and from my Hara directed the energy through my hands and visualized the dissolution of the hemotoma.

To my perception and amazement it dissolved almost immediately and the sub-cranial bleeding ceased. At the same moment both his heartbeat and respiration slowed and he began to moan. In about five minutes he was fully awake and complaining of the pain the wound was causing him. There was a collective sigh of relief from both the Russians and the Imperial officials present.

The Crown Prince called for brandy but I forbade it; instead I called for green tea and administered a small dosage of morphine to assist in alleviating the pain. I was then informed that two trains had left Tokyo, one containing the Imperial envoy Kitashiwakawa and numerous other Imperial officials. The other contained the Emperor's Imperial physician and the entire staff of the Tokyo Imperial Medical University. They arrived a number of hours later and he was examined by all.

It was determined simply that he had suffered a mild concussion from the blow and feeling that further explanation of his condition would be fruitless, I concurred. I was profusely thanked by both the Imperial physician and the Imperial envoy and sent on my way.

The next day I was invited to the Imperial Russian presence and thanked by the Crown Prince himself who presented me with a small dagger and 1000 gold rubles for my fee. I attempted to decline the offer saying how embarrassed I was that such a horrible thing had occurred in my country.

He, in a very friendly but nevertheless imperious manner, refused my refusal to accept and told me that it was only a small way to express his gratitude. I then accepted and inquired if he needed anything in the way of medical or other attention. He informed me that he was being overly cared for and truly nothing else was needed or in fact would be welcome. We chatted for a few more moments on inconsequential things such as the weather and the beauty of Lake Biwa and I politely withdrew.

I was immediately grabbed by the police commandant and escorted to the room of the Imperial envoy Kitashiwakawa who expressed the Emperor's personal thanks for my quick attention to the Crown Prince and indicated that he would be in contact with me after I had returned to Tokyo.

Subsequently, a few weeks after my return, I was summoned by two of the Imperial bodyguards and accompanied into his presence.

After I was accompanied to his audience room, he expressed his gratitude and then to my complete and utter shock the Emperor himself entered dressed casually in Western garments and personally himself expressed his gratitude. Whereupon I was presented with a small tea service from the Nara period and three embroidered silk kimonos, one for myself and one for my mother and father, a small letter signed by the Emperor himself and a purse containing 5000 British sovereigns. This money combined with the Crown Prince's gift I used to found my small clinic a little later.

After taking tea and refreshment with the Emperor and envoy, the Emperor withdrew and I was offered a position on the staff of the Imperial Medical College. I explained to minister Kitashiwakawa that there were certain aspects about my medical practice which were traditional rather than modern and this might cause a conflict with the other staff and professors. Though pressing me a few times to accept, the envoy was relieved at my refusal.

I am sure that I had been thoroughly investigated before this audience and that mention perhaps had been made of my traditional inclinations toward healing which would not have been generally accepted by the Medical University staff. After much polite small talk I was dismissed and readily withdrew. I was shown to one of the Imperial carriages and returned home.

Unfortunately, just as I was leaving the Imperial grounds, my stomach, responding to the excitement and awe of having met the Emperor in person, insisted on emptying its contents to the politely concealed amusement of my guards. They did comment however, that should they have had an audience, they probably would have done the same thing, but most likely in the Imperial presence. Mentally I thanked all the Buddhas and Kami that that had not occurred in my case.

A few weeks later a number of members of the Imperial envoy on Kitashiwakawa's staff consulted me and later a number of other notables from the Court as well as their families. This greatly gratified me.

After the attempted assassination, our country had a great outpouring of sympathy and apology which was most graciously accepted by the Crown Prince whose sympathy for the Emperor's grief was even reported in the Russian press. I was most pleased at my small part in the affair. I am also happy that the Crown Prince recovered quickly without further incident or any disablement.

Translation of a Lecture by Dr. Usui to 15 of His Graduating Students on 11 June 1916 in the Garden of his home.

Usui writes...

In dealing with the general public, one must first have the obligation to be grave and not give in to frivolity. One must never, and I truly mean never, show oneself to one's patient after consuming even the tiniest amount of alcohol. If one smokes tobacco one must not do so when counselling with a patient.

One must not be seen with questionable companions or seeking about for loose women. One should not be flamboyant in one's dress, so as to call unfortunate attention to oneself. One's home life should be above reproach, even when the servants are not present. One should not inappropriately comport oneself in the presence of the servants for you know it is said that a servant's tongue is like a dagger; it can stab in many directions.

It is said that in the days of Ieyasu Tokugawa there was a certain general who had a stomach complaint which afflicted him constantly. This unfortunate man would punish the mistakes of his subordinates with extreme severity. One day he made a small mistake and the Shogun immediately sentenced him to death. In amazement, he asked the Shogun why such a small mistake had caused his death. The Shogun replied, "Sir, I am only following your example."

The general immediately repented and was forgiven his small error, by the Shogun. Therefore, take this into consideration and hold it in mind.

Also another story comes from that time about giri. ('Giri' translated from Japanese to English means: "debt", "obligation", "responsibility", "contract", or "vow".) A woman lived on the lands of a Daimyo and wove rice straw shoes for her living. Every year she would ask the Daimyo the price for some rice straw. Every year he would say, "Simply take it." She would say, "No, I make a profit from it and it is your rice straw." He would say, "But I have no use for it." She would reply, "Nevertheless it belongs to you and it is not mine." Then he would chuckle, and demand a small price. When she had made the shoes and collected her profit, she would then go to his steward and pay the amount.

She was taken sick one year and could not work. As she was a widow supporting her grandchildren, the family was in serious trouble. She was very surprised when the Daimyo appeared with food and a bag of coins, at her door. She inquired why he had come and was told, "Honoured Aunt, over many years you have served me faithfully, insisting on giving me what is my right although I did not want to take it. You have more than fulfilled the obligation of a loyal subject to your Lord. Would that all Samurai be as scrupulous in discharging their obligations. Therefore, now you must let me as your Lord discharge my obligation to you, or I shall have no face."

The woman understanding this, gratefully accepted the food and coins. She recovered and served him faithfully many more years.

As the Christians say, her Daimyo recognized that she had been faithful in a small thing to him, so he was faithful to her. Therefore, let us take this to heart and hold it in our minds that even the smallest obligation is important to fulfil. If we do not fulfil small obligations how then can we be willing to fulfil greater and more important obligations.

Many people today would think the woman's act was senseless. If she could acquire free rice straw, she was stupid to have paid for it. She would have lost some profit. Let me tell you she was not stupid. She honestly fulfilled an obligation that she recognized whether the Daimyo considered it important or not was not the question. She considered it important. Even though it was his straw it was her obligation. It would have been most unlikely that he would even have taken notice of the straw. He obviously did not care about it and asked her to take it. But she knew better than he her obligation, as the straw was his. He had paid his tenants to grow it for its rice. He had taken the rice, the straw remained but was also his. She had no right to it. She honoured his rights to the straw. And although he would have burned the straw to clear the field, it was his straw to burn and not hers. She recognized his right and her obligation and like an ethical person fulfilled that obligation.

Even if he was not mink, but greedy, he still would have fulfilled his obligation to the latter; if he had not, it would have become apparent to everyone that he had not, and he would have lost a great deal of face. Instead, they both gained face through their acts. She gained face by paying, he by fulfilling his obligation.

This is the way that society should function. When every individual fulfils his obligation, there is little need for civil law or criminal law. There would be little need for police, for when people can recognize their obligations and be set on fulfilling them, there are no disputes. That is why from the year 1616 to the year 1867 peace reigned and prosperity abounded in Japan. By the example of the Tokugawa Shoguns people fulfilled their obligations to one another, government, and Emperor.

THE OBLIGATIONS OF A HEALER

Usui writes....

Now to go on about the obligation of a healer. We have essentially said that before fulfilling one's obligation to one's patients one has to fulfil one's primary obligations. If one does not then it should be clearly evident that they do not have the proper inclination to be a healer. So now that this has been dealt with let us go on.

I have talked about moral conduct in general, but in particular moral conduct is incumbent upon the healer. This particular moral conduct is even more important and binding than the general moral conduct our society prescribes.

The first is: One must never, and this is absolute, knowingly take any action that will cause harm to one's patient. That is why it is much better not to act according to allopathic discipline prescribing a treatment unless one is absolutely certain of benefit to the patient. One has the certainty that if one uses Reiki on behalf of the patient, one can cause no harm. Whereas the incorrect allopathic or Chinese remedy could worsen the condition. One has the obligation to act if one knows how, and refrain from acting, an even stronger obligation, if one is not certain of the benefits of the treatment.

Now do you want to hear a very amusing story? A young Western widow came to me complaining that her menses had ceased. She had been to another doctor who had tried a number of remedies to bring on the menses without success. Her husband had been dead over a year. I began to question the girl thinking she was exhibiting all the symptoms of an early pregnancy. She said this could not possibly be as her husband had been dead for over a year.

I sent her home, consulted all my books on gynaecology and even borrowed some from a friend. I saw her two weeks later and her womb was filling with fluid and was imitating a normal pregnancy. I decided to question her some more. Being careful to be exceedingly tactful as she was a Western woman, we got to the point of sexual intercourse. Oh, yes, she had engaged eleven times over the past year but was suffering under the delusion that women could only become pregnant from their husbands because that was the way in which God had ordained it.

I explained carefully to her that was not the case; she insisted that might be so for Japanese but was not true for Christian Westerners. I asked her to wait in my waiting room while I called a Western colleague and to his unrestrained amusement explained her peculiar belief. He agreed to see her and she and her mother returned to California and were never seen again in Japan. Since she was a healthy young woman, I assume the birth was normal and both she and her mother were proved wrong.

It is interesting for me to say here that I have never had a case quite like hers again, but I have treated a number of Western female patients who until I explained it to them, did not connect the act of sexual intercourse with their condition of pregnancy. I also examined a young Western man who frankly disclosed to me that he believed that kissing could result in pregnancy. I explained to him that whereas kissing might lead to the act, that kissing alone could not impregnate a girl.

I have also treated five young Western ladies who also believed that kissing was the primary cause of pregnancy. On questioning them I found that their mothers had all told them this in order to discourage the practice.

But to return to my patient and her original story. Had I prescribed a laxative or attempted to bring on menses by other Western practices or Chinese herbs, I could well have caused a miscarriage, the subsequent death of the fetus and perhaps haemorrhage and death of the mother, but I refrained from treatment until I could research her problem, and then spent the time to judiciously question her and thus discovered the primary cause of her condition.

I could either regale or bore you with many more anecdotes of this kind but I will not for it is time for us to go on.

OBLIGATION TO MEDICINE BUDDHA

Usui writes....

We have talked about obligation and the necessity for its application in daily life as well as in the practice of the healing arts. There are two primary obligations I wish to mention. And for us they should be those two obligations that are the most important in our lives.

The first: Our obligation as healers to Medicine King Buddha. From Medicine King Buddha all healing energy, whether allopathic, naturopathic, homeopathic, or spiritual, flows. He is the fountain from which flow the streams of solace, healing, and comfort for all beings. He is the bright noonday sun whose gentle rays dispel darkness, ignorance, and suffering. He is the moon whose gentle luminosity brings solace and comfort to the careworn and show travellers in the darkness of night that path wherein they should walk. He is the great mountain of compassion who can be seen by all beings from wherever they look. To behold him they must simply turn their eyes to him.

He is the ocean of wisdom who bathes those who would plunge into him with knowledge and instruction. He is the perfect enlightened energy whose lapis lazuli radiance sheds its gentle glow throughout Samsara. It is he who will lead us by the practice of the discipline of healing and through the merit gained therefrom bestows perfect enlightenment. He is our guide on the path and we have no surer guide among Gods or men. He can only work for our benefit, not our harm, engaging only in actions which lead to assistance and healing.

Looking therefore at the face of this sublime benefactor, we know then our obligation to him, one that can be repaid only in achieving his state of perfect enlightenment, that we too may be such supreme benefit as is he.

Now the second obligation, but a secondary obligation which is part of the first and is as important: Since the time of Buddha Shakyamuni the great masters have handed down to us knowledge which is beyond value and concept. If all the riches in the three thousand-fold universe were to be gathered together and placed in a balance, it would be like a grain of sand compared to this entire earth; that is its value. Yet Medicine King, Amitabha, Shakyamuni, through the masters of the lineage have freely made this available to us. My own teacher Watanabe Bonze, my medical professors, the village doctor whose kindness so inspired me, whether they are aware of it or not, are all masters of this great lineage of healing and worthy of the respect that would be given to Medicine King Buddha himself.

Now I am not saying this to you expecting you to fall at my feet in abject devotion, for you have all treated me well, and I find nothing lacking in your devotion, and respect, nor in the financial support you have chosen to bestow upon me for your teaching. You are good students and all have been so since you have been with me. I am telling you this to make you aware that anyone, your teachers at university, even those with the round devil eyes (Westerners) and strange coloured hair, are all of this same healing lineage.

Most certainly with only one exception I know of, those from the West are not aware of this, but many of them erroneously believing that it was their Christian deity and not Medicine King Buddha, who has inspired them to enter the healing professions, and not only that but to travel a great distance in uncomfortable sailing vessels to help us learn their techniques of healing for our benefit.

Many of my colleagues ask why I take time and money to teach young dullards like yourselves. It is simple. I cannot take even a hair's breadth of my fortunes and possessions into my next life. Some day I will appear before the Lord of Death, for judgement and then my next life will be determined. Since I can't take any of my possessions with me, and since he is known to be incorruptible anyway, I cannot pay him a bribe, but I can show him my honour and my students. You are my true wealth. This is true. But of course this is not the only reason I am teaching you.

I believe in what I am saying and that belief alone determines my action. After today you will go to different places and do different things. I may see some of you again, others I may never see. But as each of you go your own way and begin healing, I ask you to remember your obligation to me to act morally, to always speak the truth, to not say things you do not mean, to say things that you mean, keep your obligation to country, to your parents, to your clan, to your patients, to your friends, to your colleagues, but more importantly than all of us, to Medicine King Buddha, for by doing so you fulfil all of your giri to me, and by doing so you will fulfil your giri to all beings.

And to all of us your teachers from Medicine King Buddha to this woolly headed old doctor, TEACH!! For then you will have truly fulfilled your obligation.

Chapter 3

'Let us set aside our outdated sectarian views and look to the essence of what we are practicing in place of the outward forms which our minds are so attached which we place so much misguided importance.'

— ***Mikao Usui***

THE REIKI PRINCIPLES

There are five training principles which were adopted by Usui from the Meiji Emperor, these precepts hold within them many teachings and ways with which to strengthen our spiritual practice in daily life.

These should not be considered rules that we need to obey, but rather, meditations worthy of contemplation. In considering these ideals and questioning our personal relationship to these simple principles we have another way to check in with ourselves. In coming back to Usui's teachings, we can align where we are at any given moment.

As suggested in the original manuscripts, these principles should be spoken once in the morning and once in the evening.

THE FIVE TRAINING PRECEPTS FOR REIKI PRACTITIONERS, BY DR. USUI

Do not get angry today

Do not worry today

Be grateful today

Work hard today (spiritual practice)

Be kind to others today

MORAL PRECEPTS FOR REIKI PRACTITIONERS, BY DR. USUI

These moral precepts were adapted by Dr. Usui. Their origins are Shin (Pure Land) Buddhism and were written by Ippen (1239-1289) and are known as "Jishu Seikai" — Precepts for the Followers of the Timely Teachings.

These precepts remind oneself of the various aspects of the spiritual path. The emphasis with these precepts is to develop mindfulness, awareness and compassionate service to all beings."

There are 26 precepts for cultivating morality:

Devoutly revere the Buddha, the Law, and the Teachers.

Do not forget the power of meditation.

Devoutly practice the mantra.

Do not engage in superfluous disciplines.

Devoutly trust the Law of Compassion.

Do not denounce the creed of others.

Devoutly promote the sense of equality.

Do not arouse discriminatory feelings.

Devoutly awaken the sense of compassion.

Do not forget the suffering of others.

Devoutly cultivate an amicable disposition.

Do not display an angry countenance.

Devoutly preserve a humble manner.

Do not arouse the spirit of arrogance.

Devoutly visualize the source of defilement.

Do not develop a sense of attachment.

Devoutly study the Law of Evanescence.

Do not arouse the sense of greed.

Devoutly examine your own faults.

Do not make comment on the faults of others.

Devoutly go on trying to influence others.

Do not forget your own proper business.

Devoutly follow the path of enlightenment.

Do not mix with frivolous pleasure seekers.

Devoutly follow the teacher's guidance.

Do not indulge in your own desires.

Aided by these precepts to the end of the world, exert yourself and do not be negligent. The activities of body, speech, and mind have as their ultimate end a single devotion to the Buddha.

CONCLUSION OF SECTION I

Dr. Usui was indeed a great man who dedicated his life

to the pursuit of healing. His methodology, insight and practice not only awakened an ancient healing art, it also seeded this way of healing for all humanity.

The inner workings of Dr. Usui's system which have not been presented within this work, offer a complete teaching on enlightenment. As practitioners in the West integrate these new concepts, perhaps a unified form of this teaching can be made more widely available.

Dr. Usui's method of healing and enlightenment is very precise in its approach.

In terms of maintaining preservation of this sacred tradition, a complete and qualified transmission must be in place, if we are to honour Usui's teachings in a way which supports clear understanding and the appropriate unfolding of this sacred art.

The Western Reiki schools, in many regards, have not all been shining examples of these ideals. With the gross misrepresentation and fragmentation of the Western Reiki System, it is no wonder that the authentic holders of Usui's System exercise some caution. Ultimately, the goal in all of this is enlightened living, healing, and benefiting others with our wisdom, words and actions. May we, like Usui all walk towards this goal for the benefit of all that lives.

SECTION TWO

Western Universal Reiki

Having explored some of Dr. Usui's material and views, this section of this book deals with the Western or Universal Reiki system.

The methods and commentary explored are designed to map the western form and the many ways Reiki can be applied in our modern times. The material ahead is indeed one perspective of the Reiki system, and it is this author's hope, that what lies ahead may illuminate the prospective student in developing 'right understanding' of Reiki.

Chapter 4

'We are all the Buddha. Truly it is only our own obscurations, our own clouded thoughts, our own non-understanding that separate us from total and complete enlightenment.'

— Mikao Usui

WHAT IS REIKI? AN OVERVIEW

Reiki is the name given to an ancient energy healing system which was developed by Dr. Mikao Usui, a Shingon Buddhist, in the late 19th Century Japan. The word itself is essentially broken down into two parts: Rei – which translates to 'spirit, mystery, holy, nature spirit' and Ki – translates to 'energy, feeling or talent'. Perhaps the best translation for Reiki is: 'Spiritual Energy or Universal Energy'.

The Universal Energy of Reiki is a particular frequency that permeates all life. Although we do not ordinarily perceive this energy on a visual level, quantum physics has been able to recognize this energy and measure its frequency. The mystics of old have known the existence of healing power since time immemorial.

Reiki is an ancient Japanese hands-on healing modality based on the transference of vital energy. Reiki is activated by touch, so applying Reiki is as simple as placing the hands on oneself or another. This transference of healing energy occurs once the individual has received an alignment to the Reiki lineage and system. This alignment is called an attunement or initiation. A Reiki teacher, someone who is qualified to give such a transmission, facilitates this attunement. Attunement or initiation into Reiki is a necessary step, as this allows an alignment with the Reiki frequency. With this alignment our energy merges with the Reiki energy and we become a conduit or channel, much like a radio being tuned to a station. With this open, the initiate has the energy available which may then be applied for healing effects to numerous situations.

Reiki is applied via the hands. The practitioners of Reiki simply place their hands on the corresponding chakras, meridians and organs, transferring healing energy to the recipient. The result is a deeply relaxing experience for both the healer and the person receiving.

No movement is required when giving a treatment and it is also not necessary to remove clothing or to fix the mind in deep focus to achieve its healing effects.

When we consider that energy is the foundation of all life, it makes sense that if we have more energy constantly available to us, the natural by-product of this is a gradual enhancement of our health and personal well-being. So, it is by the transference of Reiki healing, there is a noticeable increase in the body's natural ability to heal itself.

AN INTELLIGENT ENERGY

Reiki is an intelligent energy. Many people liken the energy to the source and all-pervading power. Many traditions have a variety of names for this power, for example: God, Buddha Mind, Nature, Universe, Great Spirit, The Force, etc. Regardless of semantics, essentially the importance lies in the notion that a higher force does permeate all existence, and that one can tap this potential through specific methods to benefit sentient beings. What this means is that when one becomes attuned to the Reiki system, there is effectively a merging of the divinity within our own spirit with that of the creative force.

To put it simply, we have a direct line to God or Buddha consciousness. Now this is not to say that once we are attuned to the Reiki energy, all our problems are solved and we no longer have any difficulties in our lives. What it does suggest is that once this alignment is made, our connection to the source of power is ignited. We then have a greater capacity to use this healing power, by introducing this to situations to heal and awaken ourselves and others. This power is creative flow, it is held together by love and is the divine intelligence manifested within you.

As we practice these methods, the doorway between our inner spirit and that divinity of the source, gradually increases. It is for this reason that Reiki can promote one's spiritual path, inner awakening, wisdom and peace.

WHO IS DOING THE HEALING?

When we are facilitating healing for another, it is important to know that we are simply conduits for healing energy. In effect, we are not the ones performing the healing, we are the instruments. One could draw the analogy of ourselves as the power cable, and the healing energy of Reiki as the electricity passing though it. As simple as this seems, it also serves as a reminder to act with humility, as we cannot fully know the possible outcomes of the healing that occurs.

This is not to negate our own part in the experience, because without being this channel the healing has no conduit to pass through. So it is that we both play a part in healing, it is a sacred union or bond between Reiki and ourselves.

WHY LEARN REIKI?

Reiki is one of the simplest yet profound healing systems known to human kind. The following are some of the many reasons why one would learn this ancient healing art.

- Reiki is a complementary therapy to traditional and Western allopathic medicine.
- Reiki assists in the healing of the physical, emotional, mental and spiritual bodies.
- Reiki is a powerful yet gentle healing art that provides the receiver and giver with additional life force. As a result, this boosts the body's natural ability to heal itself.

- Reiki summons the potential for growth and spiritual development in a being.
- Reiki is always safe and provides spiritual nourishment and protection to the attuned person.
- Reiki requires no previous religious practice or spiritual traditions for one to benefit.
- Reiki evokes the highest potential for healing and self-empowerment.
- Reiki is an effective tool to heal oneself and others including psychological, spiritual and emotional issues.
- Reiki can be learnt by anyone regardless of previous experience, education or healing ability.
- Reiki can be used for first aid, to heal animals, children and anyone who is out of balance.
- Reiki enhances insight, creative flow and higher understanding of oneself and one's perception.
- Reiki is a simple tool to reduce stress and enhance inner peace.
- Reiki training is simple and easy to learn and requires little effort to achieve positive results.

Chapter 5

The seeker who has confidence in the way will go beyond the way and find the end of suffering. The seeker who goes beyond the way enlightens the world, just as the moon shines as it passes from behind the clouds.'

— ***The Dhammapada***

THE ATTUNEMENT PROCESS

Where one develops the ability to facilitate Reiki is in the attunement process. It is the foundation for bestowing the empowerment in using the hands for healing.

The attunements or initiations of traditional Reiki are an integral and essential part of Reiki. It is these alignments, which make the connection possible with the Reiki energy.

The process of initiation into Reiki is an exact science, or if you like, a formula. This is why it is essential if we wish to gain a complete and pure connection with the Reiki energy, we need the correct empowerments from a qualified Reiki teacher.

Because Reiki is an oral transmission from teacher to student, one cannot simply read a book on Reiki or surf the websites on the internet, and as a result have the ability to facilitate Reiki healing. It is not enough to have an intellectual understanding of how it works to achieve lasting results, nor will wishful thinking bring lasting results. We need the empowerments from someone who knows how.

So how do the Attunements work? The initiations are an ancient formula of energy renewal. The keys to these ancient formulas lie in the Reiki symbols, which if drawn and visualized in the correct sequence by an empowered teacher, will effectively create this pathway in the recipient. Further to this, to have lasting results, there are a number of factors which need to be met, for an effective alignment, these are as follows:

THE FACILITATOR (REIKI TEACHER)

1. That the initiating teacher has an unbroken lineage in the Reiki system. What this means is, that the initiating teacher must have received the empowerment to the third degree, (the level which empowers the individual to teach and initiate Levels I and II).
2. That the initiating teacher has been empowered from a Senior Reiki teacher, (one who has the ability to teach and empower teachers).
3. At the minimum level, the initiating teacher needs to facilitate the four separate attunements of Level I for a permanent and lasting result.

If these factors are met, and provided the initiating teacher has the correct procedures and carries these out appropriately, then the full alignment to the Reiki energy will occur every time.

This is always the case, regardless of belief or intention on behalf of the recipient.

For an individual to have this alignment, one only needs an energy system to qualify.

The initiation procedure works beyond concept, intention or belief system.

As described by Dr. Usui, one does not need to add new things to the Reiki system. The system is complete in itself.

FACTORS OF REIKI ALIGNMENT

The following are some of the factors involved with the attunement process and its results on the human energy system.

- The initiation process works specifically on the chakra system, creating a new pathway of energy, which is distributed throughout the whole body with touch being its direct activation.
- The attunement process uses the structural energetics of the body (the chakras and the central channel), as a pathway for healing energy.
- The attunement process uses the pathway of the central channel. The result of initiation affects the seven chakras and has a direct effect on the whole of our being, physically, emotionally, mentally, psychically and spiritually.
- This new pathway also operates independently of the chakra system.

What this means is our own ego, mind, emotions and feeling cannot disrupt this flow.

This is why the recipient does not need to hold any mental focus or attention for this energy to manifest. This is also true of facilitating Reiki on oneself or another. All one needs to do, once attuned, is to place ones' hands on the body and the Reiki energy will flow. One could say, once attuned, we are constantly on 'automatic'.

One can also perform self-healing when one is ill, emotionally upset or distressed, these feelings have no effect upon the transmission of Reiki energy. In healing others, it makes sense to be in balance first, however even in these circumstances, the healing energy being transferred to another comes through the facilitator first, so both receive healing energy at the same time.

The very act of facilitating Reiki, elevates one's mood, relaxation and stability whenever the hands are placed upon oneself or another.

- The Reiki energy also does not switch off when we change our state of consciousness. For example when we fall asleep, perhaps giving ourselves Reiki, the energy still transmits. It is not dependant upon our conscious awareness for it to work effectively. Students can actually do a lot of personal healing whilst asleep. By placing the hands on the body when comfortable in bed, this practice not only promotes restful sleep, but the subtle healing of the body as well.
- Once the student has received the four attunements of Reiki, this alignment can never be lost or taken away; it remains as a permanent alignment for the rest of the person's physical life.

Essentially Reiki is activated by touch, so as long as the hands are in contact with the body, the energy begins to flow, transmitting healing energy to whatever is required in the given situation.

As a general guide, the Reiki energy will also activate within 7 centimetres off the body, however, the energy also activates in a variety of ways and can be experienced when the hands are not in contact with the body. For example: whilst doing meditation, Tai Chi or Chi Kung, relaxing or simply enjoying a creative task.

Reiki is essentially a hands on modality, so it is preferable to proceed in your session with both hands on yourself or the person you are working on.

RIGHT PROCEDURE, RIGHT OUTCOME

The importance of having the correct initiation procedures can be likened to a chemical formula. For example, the Reiki Attunement process is like the formula H_2O, which translates as water. Now if we change this formula slightly to H_2O_2, in chemistry we get hydrogen peroxide.

This was only a slight change with a dramatic effect. Similarly, if we change the attunement procedures and introduce new symbols and/or new procedures outside the Reiki system, we cannot be certain of the outcome. This is why it is essential to have the correct alignment in the traditional system and to perform these procedures correctly every time.

There are many Reiki systems out there, and many initiation sequences being published both in books and over the Internet. These sequences are not intended for anyone to experiment with. As mentioned previously, one needs the correct alignment and training to be most effective in their transmission. Without this, one could liken it to performing surgery without any expertise or training. The danger of proceeding without the necessary understanding and guidance from someone who knows, is often a hit and miss affair. It is one thing to tinker with such sacred teachings on oneself, but it is quite another to tamper with another individual's path.

It is also important to note here, that there are many variations of the attunement procedures. Some vary greatly from the traditional initiations, and others vary only slightly in procedure and content.

Depending upon the person facilitating the attunements and the procedures used, outcomes vary. Just because one attunement procedure differs from another does not mean it will not work. The majority of the time, some ability is transferred; however, the degree of potency and effectiveness of these procedures differ depending upon the factors mentioned previously. Certainly procedure, lineage and right motivation play an integral part in the transference of an effective healing ability.

RESULTS OF INITIATION

Purification: Purification occurs throughout the Reiki System and roughly translates as a clearing of past blockages, obstacles to happiness, toxins, and dysfunctional patterns within our being.

Some purification can be felt as various aches and pains, headaches, nausea, dizzy spells, diarrhoea, and feeling spacey. These experiences are often only temporary and soon pass.

One does not usually experience all of these symptoms and sometimes not at all. However, it is comforting to know that although uncomfortable at the time, these symptoms are a result of the Reiki initiation and are generally a temporary experience.

We may experience mood swings and both old and new emotional pain.

Again, this is often not a dramatic experience, and passes gently. The thing to remember is that if you are not experiencing these purifications of the body and mind, don't worry. It does not mean that it is not working, it just depends on how the Reiki energy is working through you. The purifications, which occur as a result of initiation, vary from individual to individual, so what we experience is a very personal thing. The majority of the time, receiving Reiki attunements is a very enjoyable and enlightening experience. The following are some of the positive experiences one may have.

Positive Experiences

When we receive this alignment to the Universal energy, we are effectively remembering who we truly are, and on a deeper level in our consciousness we recognize this. Many people report a feeling of 'coming home', or that the feelings that arise have a familiarity to them, as if they are remembering an ancient part of themselves. With ongoing use of the Reiki energy in one's daily life, these emotions and feelings naturally manifest more and more, and we become attuned to this.

The reasons for these changes in the way we view ourselves and our reality, is due to the new 'lens' which the initiations ignite within. We are all veiled in so many ways through our past conditioning. The Reiki initiations remove some of these veils, enabling us to see past our small views and truly to see what was always there.

Part of this continued alignment, often translates to a greater sensitivity to the needs of our body and mind. Many people report that the need for various crutches like tobacco, coffee and alcohol changes in them. They have noted a much lower tolerance for the substances which create imbalance, and a greater desire for life sustaining foods and positive habits which promote health and vitality.

This can also translate as a deeper knowing of what our body requires for balance.

The Reiki energy creates a pathway to our inner knowing, and this means knowing what is best for us on the level of our body, speech and mind.

Chapter 6

Medicine King Buddha spoke to me and said I was a physician as he was, and that it would be my job, my mission, to make a synthesis of both teachings.'

— ***Mikao Usui***

PREPARING FOR A REIKI I CLASS

Once you make the commitment to attending a Reiki class with your chosen teacher, certain forces begin to come into play. Quite often people experience subtle changes or shifts within and around themselves. In a way, the deeper part of yourself, your unconscious mind and spiritual mind is preparing for the attunements. Initiation translates as 'doorway', and it is indeed a doorway which you pass through, into a new alignment with the Universal Source.

In making the decision to learn Reiki, the energy begins to meet with you and raises your personal vibratory level. Many people report that they can feel subtle sensations in their hands and body even before turning up to the workshop. It is the Divine Intelligence of the Reiki energy working with you, removing obstacles from your personal growth and healing.

Other experiences may translate in the dream state, with dreams occurring, which can be vivid and highly symbolic.

Reiki I, The First Degree

Reiki I is the first level in the traditional Western Reiki System. The first degree or beginner's level offers many benefits, and of all the levels offers the most dramatic connection. This is because it is the first time the initiate receives the Reiki Alignment with the Universal energy.

In Reiki I there are four initiations. These initiations gradually open the individual to the full capacity of the level one energy, and these four separate attunements highlight specific areas of the body.

THE RESULTS OF THE FOUR REIKI I ATTUNEMENTS

Attunement 1

- Creates a temporary alignment with the Universal energy.
- Highlights the Crown and Heart chakras and the connection between the two.
- Highlights the palm chakras.
- Both inner and outer energy merge and this pathway is extended through the hand chakras.

Attunement 2

- This initiation works on the heart/thymus and palm chakras.

- Widens the recipient's channel from the Universal energy source.

Attunement 3

- This initiation, although being the same as the second, deepens the connection in the heart/thymus and palm chakras and further expands the channel within the individual.
- Enhances and expands the benefits of the second initiation.

Attunement 4

- This final initiation works specifically on the pituitary and pineal glands and seals the recipient with the first degree Reiki permanently.
- At completion of the fourth initiation the individual has a complete alignment with the Universal energy and this can never be lost or hindered.
- This initiation completes the previous three initiations and aligns the recipient permanently to Reiki healing energy.

PRE-ATTUNEMENT GUIDELINES

As a general guide, it is suggested to prepare oneself before a Reiki class.

It is best to do what feels right for you in regard to this, as we all have different needs.

The following are some useful guidelines which you may wish to engage in. They are presented here to assist you in setting the stage for a wholesome experience.

- Avoid taking any substances that may cloud the mind such as caffeine, heavy foods, cigarettes, alcohol or recreational drugs. These substances have a direct effect on the energy system and generally hinder higher resonance energy flow.
- Keep the days preceding and the evenings between the workshop, quiet and passive where possible. Often, before and within the class environment, we go into a deep and nurturing space. It is best to support this by keeping the space we hold outside of the workshop, nurturing and still. This assists in maintaining the thread of the day to day experience.
- Nurture yourself. Set time aside to simply be with yourself. Do something that gives you pleasure, a walk on the beach or in nature or even a candle-lit bath. You may wish to utilize this time to reflect on your life to date and to think about how you might integrate what you have learnt in the workshop so far. A Reiki workshop is a unique time for reflection and change.

PURIFICATION AND THE ATTUNEMENTS

Occasionally, once having received the attunements, an individual may experience a cleansing and detoxifying process. This process is most heightened during the workshop and the following three days. The suitable effect may also be experienced for a period of 21 days. Some of these are as follows:

- A short cold or flu just after the workshop.

- Headaches or mild nausea.
- Fatigue or heightened energy.
- Hot flushes, dizziness or sweating.
- Types of emotional releases such as crying or laughter.
- Various aches or pains due to releasing of blockages both energetically and physically.

As we are purifying these obstacles, it is important to consider that the process of purification is a process, and therefore will pass. The degree of how we experience this will vary from person to person. This is largely dependent upon our own personal path and how much work we have done on ourselves. Generally speaking, if we have led unhealthy lives, have many unresolved issues and project negative and destructive thoughts and views, then the degree of this purification will be heightened.

As you are moving through this process, it is highly recommended to continue practicing your self-healing treatments. In giving yourself Reiki, your hands on sessions will enhance this healing process, and support you in your newfound ability.

It is also not uncommon for our symptoms to temporarily increase, during this process.

The reason for this is due to the accelerated rate of healing. If you are processing then you may try a different approach to your healing. You may give yourself Reiki in small but regular doses. For example: 5 or 10 minutes every few hours, or instead 1 hour once a day, it is really up to you and a question of how much time you wish to make for self-healing.

It is especially important to continue this process for the 21 days proceeding a Reiki I class.

It is during this time that we begin to form a solid and stable relationship with the Universal energy of Reiki.

It is often said, that if you are experiencing joy and bliss, then this is good. If you are experiencing purification and discomfort, then this is also good. It is all good, because healing is taking place.

SELF-HEALING

'If you don't take care of your body, where will you live?'

— Unknown

Of the many things Reiki can offer, self-healing is perhaps the most important of all. Each time we apply Reiki to ourselves we are furthering the pathway to our healing. This is not such a difficult task, as we instinctively have our hands-on our own body throughout the course of a day. Reiki is a natural thing to do. We see this so often. What do we do when we hit ourselves on the thumb with a hammer (besides hopping around making a lot of noise)? We hold it.

With a Mother or a sick or upset child, it is her hands providing the healing touch, by holding and comforting the child.

It is said that touch communicates more in five seconds than five minutes of talking.

So, it makes sense that if we hold ourselves with full alignment to the Universal energy, we will naturally be transmitting, not only self-healing but self-love. Reiki is a great way to become reacquainted with ourselves, to touch and nurture ourselves.

In the words of Mrs. Takata (the third Reiki master of the Western lineage): "A little Reiki is better than none at all"; so whether it is five minutes or one hour, there is always some benefit. The approach with Reiki is much like homeopathy; it is better to do a little on a regular basis rather than a lot, say, once a month. A mini session can simply comprise five minutes on yourself before you get out of bed in the morning, or by placing your hands on yourself after a meal to aid your digestion.

If we are approaching Reiki as a chore, for example: "Oh, I have to do my practice today", then we have the wrong view. The important thing to remind ourselves is that our hands have an additional role to play. These are not just hands that can do amazing things, but are instruments of creating healing, pleasure and balance.

In addition to your Reiki mini sessions, you may wish to give yourself a full treatment once a day or weekly. This process is the same as giving a full treatment on another, instead corresponding the hand positions to yourself.

A self-healing treatment can also take the form of working specifically with one of a number of the chakras, or working on holographic models of the body, i.e.: the feet (reflexology).

If you are feeling stressed, lie down or sit back and place your hands over your eyes or on the back of your head. Reiki is a very simple concept, if something hurts, then reach for your hands before you reach for an aspirin.

It is also important to consider going to the area of concern, early in the piece. Don't wait for a headache to become a migraine before you use your Reiki. The sooner 'hands on' healing is activated, the sooner Reiki can work its magic.

Naturally with any healing, whether it be self-healing or healing others, we need to use Reiki with common sense. If a situation calls for medical advice and treatment, we should always follow this. Reiki is a complementary adjunct to western medicine, so with this in mind, ideally we use the best of both worlds.

HELPING OTHERS. HOW MUCH REIKI?

A common concern for practitioners is how much Reiki to give in any given situation. The length of a treatment and the time between sessions is largely dependant on the individual concerned, and the time available to the practitioner and the recipient. Generally, sessions last anywhere from thirty minutes to one and a half hours. The length of time between a session can be anywhere from one day to a week. If a person has a major illness or would like to work intensively on an issue, then it is suggested that four treatments are given over four consecutive days. The results of these sessions are then assessed. In some cases, one may not see the breakthrough of a problem until the third or fourth day. The reasons for this vary; however, each progressive session builds on the previous one, thereby enhancing the capacity of Reiki-healing taking place within the body.

Committing to a number of sessions is sometimes a big task for a prospective client, and as a practitioner, it is important to explain the healing process in terms of the recipient's needs.

If such a commitment is made, then one should supplement this commitment by a reduced rate for on-going consultations.

WHAT DOES ONE EXPERIENCE IN FACILITATING REIKI?

Whether you are conducting Reiki for yourself or another, there are a variety of experiences that can be perceived.

The most common of these experiences are:

1. A feeling of heat or warmth in the hands.
2. Tingling or pulsing up or down the arms and in the body.
3. Cold or cool energy running through the hands.
4. The cessation of mental chatter, and increased calm.
5. Deep relaxation.
6. Visual impressions, seeing colours, lights or images.
7. Hands feeling drawn to an area.
8. Hands feeling repelled from an area.
9. Hands feeling like they are stuck or glued in an area.
10. Hands feeling like they are a few inches inside the area that is being worked on.
11. An occasional sharp or dull pain in your hands or arms.
12. A slight vibration in the hands or arms.

All of the above phenomena are natural by-products of working with the Reiki energy and experiences vary from person to person. The important thing to remember is that these experiences are a result of engaging with Universal energy and, therefore, it is not essential to interpret these kinds of experiences.

As a practitioner gains greater experience, these sensations can open up information regarding the client's situation or what is required with regards to his/her healing. It does take time and practice to accurately interpret what each of these sensations mean for the individual concerned. Unfortunately, it is not all black and white; each sensation, symptom or experience can have countless meanings, interpretations and causes. So it is best not to leap to conclusions regarding an individual's needs.

Unless one is licensed to do so, one does not prescribe or diagnose a client's condition.

METAPHYSICS, A POTENTIAL BLIND SPOT FOR HEALERS

Our physical mind loves to have sensational experiences and although this can be a comforting confirmation that something is actually happening, it has no bearing on the result or effectiveness of one's healing ability. Often in Reiki courses, when other group members share experiences, we naturally compare with each other, how amazing, sensational or fantastic each person's experience is. Whatever you experience is unique and perfect for you in that moment. The art of Reiki is simplicity, so the less we involve our physical minds, the better.

There is also a danger in prescribing a particular meaning for a sensation. For example, heat meaning repressed anger or emotional pain. The danger in such generalizations lies in the practitioner placing their interpretation on the person receiving the healing. This response may not necessarily have relevance or meaning for the person concerned. As practitioners of Reiki, one should offer advice which is fairly neutral, so as not to influence a client's view.

Metaphysical causations for physical sensations are incredibly general, and more often than not bear little meaning to the cause of a person's symptoms. This is not to say that metaphysics have no place in healing. The point is that some practitioners can use these views as a general form of diagnosis, and if not qualified to give diagnosis, can influence a client regarding their actual condition. It is for this reason that cause and effect illustrations are not presented within this book. Hypothetically, when such metaphysical rules are put in place, a practitioner may simply say: 'Oh, you have a sore lower back, that's because you have repressed anger towards your father.' Whereas the real reason may be that the client injured their back in a motor vehicle accident some months previously. Such a response can leave the client, disempowered and result in the practitioner looking for the wrong approach to healing that person's complaint.

The use of metaphysics has its place in healing, but a word of warning: don't allow these concepts to cloud your judgement. Each healing situation is unique and we need to approach our healing sessions with a clear view, free of concepts.

HOW PEOPLE RESPOND TO REIKI

The ways in which a person responds to a session are many and varied. A common experience is that a session will take the recipient into a deeply relaxing space, they may even fall asleep. In others, it can bring suppressed emotions to the surface. If a person does need to cry, gently nurture them and keep applying the energy. It does not mean that you have done something wrong if a person is crying, it is the result of Reiki working on the emotions as a form of release. Tears are a way to purify blockages and emotional pain, as well as de-toxing within the physical body. Reiki is a nurturing gift, and it can heal in so many ways.

If a person has a large emotional release, be caring, but stable and ask them to breathe through it. You may even breathe with them. Breathing is one of the most effective ways to move through old emotional pain. As a practitioner you can offer a shoulder to cry on and an ear to listen. If they don't want to talk about it, that's OK. If we are not trained in counselling or basic psychology, sometimes it is better not to put on the therapist's hat. Be there for the person, be real and be caring, as this is often all a person needs to feel safe and accepted in their emotions.

HANDS-ON SESSIONS

Traditionally, Reiki follows a sequence for applying the hands upon another person. This is in order to cover the major areas of energy flow, as well as energizing the major organs and energy centres of the body. This systematic approach works on the premise of twelve positions on the front of the body and twelve positions on the back of the body. (Schools vary in this approach.)

The hand positions are a way to facilitate a general healing, and to boost the life force and vitality of the recipient. The hands are usually left in these positions for anywhere from three to five minutes, with the whole session taking approximately one to one and a half hours.

CHECKLIST FOR HANDS-ON HEALING

The following are some basic guidelines to facilitate a healing at the Reiki I level.

1. Gather information from the recipient regarding their needs.

   Ask: Have you had a Reiki Session before? If not, briefly explain the process.

   Ask: Is there anywhere that you require healing?

   Once you have a general idea of what they require, ask them to close their eyes and relax.

2. *Centering procedure*: Place your hands on your heart and close your eyes.

   Focus your intent for a brief moment. Imagine yourself being a vessel for the Universal energy and that you are now clear and present to begin the session.

3. Having affirmed this, seal your Thymus chakra by placing your hands front and back of the thymus and visualize a blue energy field.

(*Please refer to establishing personal boundaries in chapter 10 for more details.*)

This establishes your personal boundaries throughout the healing procedure.

4. In your own way commence the session, following the step by step approach of applying Reiki to the body.
5. Once you feel the healing is complete, wash your hands and seal your Thymus chakra by placing your hands in the same position as step 3. This disconnects you from the recipient's energy field.
6. Gently bring the person around and share your experiences.

   Be sure not to interpret or diagnose their condition, we simply share what we sensed in the session.

GENERAL GUIDELINES FOR GIVING A REIKI SESSION

- Be sure to remove any pets from the room, your client may be allergic to cats or dogs and animals have a tendency to disrupt a session.
- If you are going to burn aromatherapy oils or incense make sure the person does not have allergies to these, if you are unsure, don't use them.
- Be sure to wash your hands before and in between clients.
- Give the person receiving the session the opportunity to ask questions.

- Make sure they are comfortable in their position, always ask, some people will keep quiet and suffer silently to be polite.
- Make sure the placement of your hands on their body is without undue pressure, ask if your touch is at a comfortable pressure.
- Try and keep contact with their body (hands on) at all times, or within 7 cm of the body between hand positions. This ensures they know where you are and can relax.
- Wear comfortable clean clothing, preferably in layers in case you get too hot.
- If you have more than two or three clients per day, be sure to change your clothes between sessions or shower where possible as a means of maintaining energetic clarity.
- Make sure your breath is fresh and don't breathe on your client's face.
- Be sure not to place your hands too close to the client's nose, ears or throat unless there is a specific reason. These areas can be uncomfortable for the recipient, especially if your hands are too heavy.
- Use tranquil music or see if your client has a particular preference of music.

FINDING A SUITABLE REIKI TEACHER AND WHAT TO LOOK FOR

Finding an appropriate teacher is often an intuitive and synchronistic experience. If you are considering a Reiki class, it does not hurt to put in your order. If you want a good Reiki teacher, it is good to do a small manifestation ritual for what you are looking for. A simple exercise is to write the qualities you are looking for in a teacher and to give a short prayer of intent for this to manifest. In a way, we are putting in our order and when the timing is right, the best teacher for you will manifest.

This process actually works. Keep in mind that we may have to wait for the right teacher, so don't let convenience and money be your only deciding factors. It can really be a mistake to look for the cheapest Reiki class on offer. Generally speaking, if you pay peanuts for Reiki you get monkeys, so be careful!

When we are investing in our spiritual lives and personal well-being, it makes sense to research well, and not to rush in blindly because we have the quick fix mentality. Getting on the spiritual path can be really exciting and people may embrace everything with such enthusiasm, they often throw out ideas like common sense and discernment. These ideas are very important, so check in with yourself to see if it all sits well within your being.

Not all teachers out there are coming from an altruistic motivation, and it is easy to be lead astray by tricksters and deceptive characters who want nothing more than to be a subservient guru, driven by ego and financial gain at your expense.

So here are a few points to look for in a teacher:

1. Check the teacher's lineage in Reiki. He/she should be able to tell you who they learnt from and their Reiki Lineage dating back to the founding teacher, Mikao Usui.

Some Reiki lineages are many legs long and may be watered down significantly by distorted views and insufficient training from their initiating instructor.

2. Ask how long they have been teaching and how long their own teacher training was.

   Do they teach regularly and do they use Reiki on themselves and others, in other words do they practice what they preach?

3. Check to see if the training you will receive is a sufficient time frame. (Approximately 14 hours for a Reiki I workshop and 12 hours for a Reiki II workshop.) Ask how many hours are devoted to hands on healing and experiential Reiki work.

4. You may wish to ask, what specific things you will cover throughout the workshop and what you will be empowered to do after the training in each level.

   (Refer to Reiki content in this chapter for a comparison.)

5. Check to see if there is any ongoing support after the training, or opportunity to practice with others after the workshop. Will the teacher be available for you after the workshop?

6. Will you receive a Certificate in Reiki upon completion?

7. Is the cost reasonable and are you supplied with a reference manual? Will you get what you paid for?

   Ask if you are able to take notes in the class or tape-record the information presented.

9. Check in with your intuitive or gut feeling. Does this person sound authentic, and are they coming from

the right motivation? Do you resonate well with this person?

10. Can the teacher send you supporting material on the workshop content and the courses available?
11. Make sure your prospective teacher recommends integration time between Reiki levels. Be wary of teachers offering combined Reiki levels or skipping levels that you have not yet completed.
12. Who will be giving the initiations at the seminar and how many initiations will you receive? (Four at Reiki I and one at Reiki II.)
13. Check to see if any symbols are taught in the Reiki levels and which ones are being taught. There should not be any symbols taught at the Reiki I level, and only three Reiki symbols taught in Reiki II. (*Refer to Reiki II symbols, chapter 10.*)
14. Has the teacher the experience to teach you? How long have they been teaching Reiki?
15. How many people does the teacher have in a single class? Will their be time set aside for self-healing and healing others?
16. What form do the classes take ? Are they over one, two, three days or are these classes spread out over a number of days or weeks?
17. Where will the seminar be held and is this practical for you?

As a guide, be wary of teachers making outrageous or extraordinary claims, and see how your ego responds to these ideas. If you are still unclear, see if the teacher is prepared to meet you personally to discuss in further detail, what will be covered throughout the workshop.

It makes sense to know with whom and what you are becoming involved with, so exercise some caution when finding a teacher. There are so many Reikis available these days, and not all systems are coming from the right motivation, methodology, understanding or integrity.

Overall, it all boils down to trusting your intuition. The person should be a living example of the things they practice. Literally, they should: 'walk their talk!'

Watch your personal expectations – most integrated teachers are not dressed in white robes and act in a holier than thou fashion. An awakened teacher is usually down to earth, realistic and normal in appearance. Be wary of sensational and over-the-top characters.

It may take time to find a good teacher and learning Reiki is not something to rush into.

Make an informed choice, and exercise common sense; when it feels right and you feel supported in your choice, these are good signs that you have found the right teacher.

When the student is ready, the teacher appears! Practice patience, as the saying goes, "good things come to those who wait."

REIKI AND MONEY

> *'There's a certain Buddhist calm that comes from having... money in the bank.'*
>
> ***— Tom Robbins***

This can be a touchy subject for many. Much of our western conditioning around spiritual traditions supports the way of the spiritual martyr, living off nothing but fresh air and good vibes. This may work as a model in some traditional eastern societies where the community supports those who take a spiritual path. However, in the West, these ideas are often not part of western people's concepts.

So it is important to charge a value to what you feel you are transmitting.

Have you ever noticed what happens when someone offers you something for free? One of the most common responses is "where's the catch? or what's wrong with it?" In the west, we have little understanding of a gift without small print attached.

On a personal note, in the years I have been teaching, I have found that if an individual has a genuine desire to learn, and that individual makes the right effort, then the means for manifesting the money necessary for a place on a workshop manifests often in an unexpected way.

It is almost like the universe hears the call and supports the individual to follow his/her healing path. This does not mean that we sit at home, relying on a sum of money to fall in our laps, we need to meet the universe half-way. Nothing happens without our direct action or involvement in the world.

If our motivation is altruistic and we are doing this for the betterment of others, and our personal unfolding, then this motivation is blessed and the universe works with us to meet our desired outcome.

In this way we strike a balance with abundance, personal value and right relationship. If we have blockages with money, then it is good to do the necessary personal growth to release these concepts. Money is energy and the way to make it flow is to be actively involved in right relationship with it.

When people have issues with fees being attached to workshops, it often comes from this form of spiritual idealism. It really comes down to the value we place on Reiki. When we consider that a few hundred dollars will give us a spiritual and practical tool, not only for self-healing but the healing of others, and that this tool will be with us till the day we die, it's not such a bad investment. Reiki is a gift to ourselves, and sometimes it is hard to receive such a gift. As modern material people, it can be hard to fathom why one would give a non-material gift such as Reiki to one's self. The answer to this lies in the following: if we value our health and if we value the ability to alleviate others' suffering, then surely such a gift is worth investing in.

When we pay money for Reiki, we are not putting a price on the unconditional spiritual power of the universe, rather we are paying for the teacher's time, expertise and energy to be there in a healing and therapeutic space.

Other systems like barter are another form of exchange, for example, swapping a massage for a Reiki or things of this nature. Other times a swap is inappropriate. Say a person who wishes to learn Reiki has an egg farm and wants to swap five thousand eggs in return for the workshop, what is the practitioner going to do with five thousand eggs? So you can see that the right kind of barter is important, for there has to be an appropriate form of exchange. Unfortunately most of us live in the material world, we need to pay bills, buy food, clothing and purchase the necessary goods for basic day-to-day living.

The saying goes: "money is the root of all evil." It is not money that is evil, money is merely a symbol and our potential evil is in fact our relationship to it.

Many people have deep-seated fears about money, that there will not be enough, that they will have too much and will need to guard it from others, etc. It's about our relationship to money, our motivation, our self worth and where we are coming from that really matters. Whatever your views are on money, take a few moments to review your relationship. Is there fear, anger, greed or other emotions related to this form of currency? Check-in with yourself; if there is an emotion, move into it. See if you can locate the reason as to why you have this response and what you can do to change it.

The bottom line is, Reiki works and the benefits are lasting, far beyond any warranty you might get for a new CD player or some other material item. Material possessions will not give you lasting peace and healing, only the sacred teachings of the Spiritual path can cultivate these gifts.

Chapter 7

'Your work is to find out what your work should be and not to neglect it. Clearly discover your work and attend to it with all your heart.'

— ***The Dhammapada***

FURTHER EXTENSIONS TO REIKI

Reiki and Pregnancy

It is a great blessing for an expectant mother, family and friends to receive Reiki during a pregnancy. There have been many documented positive experiences where Reiki has been particularly helpful in pregnancy and during labour.

Reiki is also very beneficial in alleviating some of the common symptoms associated with pregnancy, such as lower back pain and morning sickness.

Daily or weekly treatments are very beneficial for mother and baby, and it is usually suggested that an expectant mother receive the four Reiki I attunements so she may give herself and her child Reiki whenever needed.

Giving the Reiki attunements to a pregnant woman is completely safe and acts as an additional blessing for the infant. Many pregnant women have attended Reiki workshops, and as a result have incorporated Reiki as part of their own self-healing and personal maintenance throughout their term. With the Mother giving Reiki to the unborn infant, there is a direct transmission of healing energy and love. This can only benefit both concerned, because, as the mother is giving Reiki to the infant in her womb, she is also transmitting healing energy to herself.

After the birth of a child, Reiki can be very effective in healing the trauma associated with birth. Some mothers have been known to give Reiki to their breasts or breast milk as the child is feeding, transmitting healing energy into the milk. Beyond the benefits of being breast fed, the child receives milk which is charged with pure life force energy and love. Reiki is also an invaluable tool for related problems in infancy, such as teething, irregular sleeping patterns (both for parents and child), feeding problems and other related problems in the early stages of development.

Reiki has also been known to assist in fertility problems by regularly directing healing energy to the sexual organs. This can be either facilitated by one's partner, or as a self-treatment procedure.

Reiki with Children

When we look at facilitating Reiki on children, the major difference is size. Having a smaller vessel (body) to work on, the session's time may decrease. As we all know, unless a child is quite ill, he/she find it difficult to remain still for extended periods of time and this becomes clear when he/she start to squirm.

One of the best ways to give your child Reiki is when they are going off to sleep, or when they are asleep. In addition to this, absent healing is another alternative to settling fears and other related emotional states. Reiki can also be effective for children experiencing nightmares. Using a simple guided meditation, which incorporates Reiki, is an effective way to settle childhood fears.

(See chapter 12 on absent healing.)

Initiating Children into Reiki

Giving Reiki attunements to a child is very beneficial, as it teaches a child from an early age to gain self-reliance and self-love. It is perhaps one of the greatest gifts one could give.

A child can be attuned to Reiki at any age. However, for a child to sit still for a physical attunement, they need to be at an age of approximately ten years old.

At the Australian Institute for Reiki Training (AIRT), we have had children as young as nine years of age who have participated in a Reiki I class accompanied by a parent. At this age, they do not take all the information in, however, this is also the case for most adults. So it is suggested, that the child reviews the course a few years later, to further the understanding and integrate the techniques and practices on a deeper level.

For children under the age of ten, the attunements are usually facilitated outside of a class environment, and the parent or guardian acts as a mentor in the basic healing procedures. When the child is ready or is mature enough, we at the AIRT invite them to participate in a Reiki I class to formalize their training.

Attunements can be facilitated with the child present, or as an absent initiation procedure. As an absent procedure, the results remain the same.

Distant attunements work especially well for:

- Children who can't sit still.
- Times when someone requests initiation and is unable to be present physically at a workshop due to health reasons or their locality.

(See chapter 18 Absent initiations.)

Working on Animals

Most domestic animals love Reiki and will often sit still long enough to receive what they require. The idea is not to force an animal to sit still, because animals are very intuitive and instinctual and know what they need in terms of receiving energy. This also works especially well for animals who are sick or dying. There are many Reiki practitioners amongst Veterinarians and other related animal health care professionals. Many of these practitioners report how the basic Reiki practices enhance the healing rate and calm the animals being treated.

Healing in the Dreamtime

As we are becoming aware, Reiki is not limited by our thoughts or our state of Consciousness.

It is the same in our sleep state. On an average we spend more than a third of our lives asleep, and the good news is, we can facilitate Reiki on ourselves whilst sleeping. As stated previously, Reiki is activated by touch and does not require our conscious effort to make it happen. When we are sleeping and have our hands in contact either with ourselves or someone else, healing energy is being transmitted.

Simply placing our hands on is not only a great way to nod off but it is also a useful time to work on our own self-healing. After a short time our hands naturally end up on our body, and during our sleep time we receive as much healing energy as is needed.

Reiki in conjunction with dream analysis, can greatly enhance dream recall and activity in the unconscious mind.

It is not uncommon for Reiki practitioners to experience heightened dream activity, and further enhancement of symbolic dreams as a result of initiation and continued Reiki practice.

Reiki naturally enhances deep rest. Many long term sufferers of insomnia and irregular sleeping patterns report the enormous benefits that Reiki has had on their sleeping patterns. Many people report that they do not need as much sleep on a regular basis, as the body is more energized and in a natural state of creative flow each day.

Research shows that individuals who are deprived of Alpha sleep have poor productivity during the day. (Alpha describes a measurement of Brain waves relating to creative states, deep awareness and relaxation. It should be noted here, that the common state of consciousness of a practitioner facilitating Reiki is in the Alpha state of consciousness. The Alpha state is the stage one enters at the tail-end of active dream-time during a night's rest.)

Whenever we are facilitating Reiki on ourselves or others, we naturally access the Alpha state and are therefore in a highly creative, vigilant and healing state of mind.

Our brains cannot help but be in this state of consciousness, which promotes healing, inspiration and insight.

REIKI AS MEDITATION

'Reiki is Wisdom and Truth.'

— ***Hawayo Takata***

When a person is either facilitating or receiving a Reiki session, the most common state of consciousness is the Alpha Level. Deep meditative and creative flow is associated with the Alpha level. So whenever we are giving or receiving Reiki, we are in fact in a state conducive to meditation. This is great news for people who say they can't meditate.

Many people commonly report a deep sense of peace and stillness as a result of Reiki healing. To work with this energy the mind naturally falls into this creative capacity. Meditation spans a variety of expressions, it is not simply sitting in full lotus position with focus on the tip of our noses. Meditation can be a walk in nature, playing a favourite sport, enjoying a creative hobby in full awareness. Although it is not completely necessary to have full awareness for Reiki to work, with practice this state of consciousness naturally begins to manifest. The more we are aware of this, the more the effects spill over into our daily lives. People who regularly meditate, often report that once they have received the Reiki attunements, they experience a greater enhancement of their meditations and are more able to sustain longer periods of stillness and awareness.

GROUP HEALING

In addition to your regular hands on sessions, group Reiki is a wonderful extension.

This is where there can be more than one person facilitating Reiki on another.

With group hands on work, we are in effect doubling our capacity to heal with an additional practitioner assisting. Now does this make Reiki better, if there is more? Not really. We are simply working in a wider capacity and transmitting healing energy at a faster rate. For example, receiving Reiki from six practitioners over a ten minute period is equivalent to a full treatment of Reiki healing from one practitioner.

Reiki comes from the highest intelligence. From this source, it goes to wherever it is needed the most, providing healing to the degree the individual can comfortably assimilate.

In a group healing, the practitioners place their hands in the positions of major energy flow. For example, one at the sides of the head, one at the upper chest, one at the lower abdomen and one practitioner at the feet. Working in this way enhances the amount of life force transmitted into the body and energy field of the recipient, and effectively balances and aligns the individual on all levels.

It is not uncommon to have the subtle reverberations of a healing, last for days or weeks. What people experience in a Reiki session varies tremendously. There are many factors to consider, such as the levels of competency of the practitioners, the recipient's level of perception, and the Karmic influences in play at the time.

LETTING GO WITH REIKI

When we receive the Reiki I initiation we are bringing a considerable amount of universal energy into our lives, so it make sense to do a little 'spring cleaning'. The 'letting go' ritual focuses on releasing our limiting beliefs and views about our lives. In this process we write on a piece of paper all the parts of ourselves that no longer serve our paths. Through this process we put a signal out to the universe, which states we are willing to let go in order to become more of who we truly are.

Letting Go Procedure: Part 1

Write on a piece of paper all the things that no longer serve you. Give thanks for the lessons that these things have given you, and state in your mind that you no longer want these in your life. Include situations and people you need to forgive.

At the end of your list, write: " I release all this now with love and sincerity, for the highest good of all concerned, I let go."

Hold the statements written on the paper, between your hands. Now imagine all of these statements as symbols or objects residing in your body. Imagine these objects leaving your body and going into the paper between your hands. Once you feel this is complete, give a prayer for the lessons you have learnt, and blow a short sharp breath between your hands. (This symbolizes the release of these issues.)

When you have completed this process, burn the page in a bowl with some sage.

Now smudge yourself, allowing the smoke to cleanse any remnants from your body and mind.

MANIFESTING WITH REIKI

Manifestation Procedure: Part 2

Write on a piece of paper all the things you wish to manifest in your life. Include situations that will serve your path and anyone's name who requires healing. Give thanks for your life and the many gifts you have. At the end of your list, write: "All this manifests now, not only for my highest good, but for the highest good of all concerned."

Hold the paper close to your body and imagine all these qualities are coming into your body, in the form of positive symbols and objects. Once you feel this is complete, offer a prayer of thanks for your life and for the opportunity to become more of your true essence.

Once you have completed this process, burn the page in a bowl with some sage.

Smudge yourself, allowing the smoke to purify and heal you. (We burn our manifestations to release our attachment to the outcome.)

Closing Procedure: Part 3

Take the ashes to a place in nature, the ocean shore, a hill or place that is special for you. Cast some of the ashes to the winds of each of the four directions, East, North, West and South, in an anti-clockwise direction.

Call all those who would help in this process, from each direction. Once the four directions have been completed, call this from above and lastly from the earth itself.

Give a final prayer of thanks for the gifts you already have in your life, and dedicate these gifts to the benefit of all life. Place the remaining ashes where you stand as a marker of the occasion. This completes the ritual.

This procedure is extremely powerful, and one will often see rapid results. We can repeat this procedure once a month, or whenever we are feeling stuck or blocked in our lives. Remember not to put fixed outcomes in your prayers or affirmations. Leave it open-ended, to allow the universe to bring this to you in the path of least resistance.

REIKI IN DAILY LIFE

We can see that Reiki has numerous applications to numerous situations.

Because Reiki is as simple as placing one's hands on oneself or another, the applications are many and varied. Incorporating Reiki into daily life is as easy as remembering that your hands have a new role to play. A little Reiki each day is better than none at all. So with this in mind, here are some helpful tips to incorporating your hands on healing from day to day.

Give yourself Reiki:

- Whilst watching a movie or TV, or send absent healing on a specific issue.
- Whilst driving your car (when a hand is free).
- When relaxing, i.e., at work with your hands behind your head in the first position.
- After finishing a meal, placing your hands on your stomach and intestines to aid in the digestion of your food.
- When walking in nature or anywhere for that matter.
- When going to sleep.
- Whenever you have a physical complaint or stress in the body.
- Whenever you have either one or both hands free.

Even if you can only do five minutes there is a connection and, therefore, some benefit.

In learning to remember that our hands are now tools for our personal empowerment, we can apply this simple principle to almost anything we can conceive. It is not necessary to limit the ways or the times in which you use Reiki. This energy is as creative and as diverse as you are. Test the boundaries and see where it takes you. There can be no harm caused using the energy alone, so as long as your personal motivation is pure, it can only lead to new and improved experiences.

Moving forward in this way, the Divine intelligence of Reiki will meet you half-way, teaching and supporting you in your journey.

Chapter 8

'Scriptures say that both wisdom lacking means and means lacking wisdom are bondage. Therefore do not abandon either.'

— ***Atisa, Bodhipathapradipa***

HEALING VERSES CURING?

When we look at the term healing, different questions come to mind. What does it mean to be healed? Does this merely involve the removal of physical afflictions or does it go deeper? Healing not only encompasses the physical being; it encompasses the whole of our consciousness. It is worth considering not only our current symptoms, but the cause as well.

Current research tells us that most modern diseases are caused by stress, poor diet and a poor personal self-image. Reiki touches every part of our being, therefore, the more we practice Reiki the greater capacity we have for health and balance. It is in this way, that many begin a healing path, either as a practitioner or simply through self-healing.

REIKI AND ALLOPATHIC MEDICINE

As described in previous sections, Reiki can be used on the physical level to complement conventional allopathic medicine. Reiki is becoming more and more popular amongst general practitioners, in hospitals and hospice-care. Because Reiki energy speeds the body's natural ability to heal itself, we find the use of Reiki to heal physical ailments is a wonderful extension.

It is important to note here that Reiki does not subscribe to being a sole method of healing, but rather, a complementary method which when used in conjunction with other therapies, can greatly assist in the rate of healing. A recipient of a Reiki session should in no way reduce or cease any medication or ignore the recommendations of a qualified health professional.

Doctors who have taken Reiki training, may use hands on during emergencies to reduce pain or calm patients who are experiencing anxiety. It has also been determined that Reiki can alter the negative effects of some drugs used in cancer treatment, and other serious illnesses. Reiki is also very popular amongst nurses, and workers in the mental health field for comforting patients who are in fear or emotional pain. At the AIRT, we have had a number of General Practitioners, nurses and mental health practitioners who have all contested to the enormous benefits of Reiki within their own practice, and in their personal self-healing.

FACTORS DETERMINING WELLNESS

In conjunction with 'hands-on' sessions it is worthy to note some of the other factors which contribute to health and well-being. Most of these ideas are based on common sense, but many of us do not consider these when we are ill or unbalanced in our lives. What we eat, how and where we sleep, and the company we keep, all determine the rate of healing.

THE ENVIRONMENT OF AN ILL PERSON

When we are ill, there is a habit to go inward, block out natural light and withdraw from people. This is not only a rapid way to become depressed, but also a recipe to remain ill. So, the environment of a room is very important in promoting health. The room of the patient should be well lit with natural light, preferably not fluorescent lighting, as well as being well ventilated. An ordered room, which is uncluttered, will also enhance positive energies. To enhance the elements of nature in a room is also a great benefit. Providing indoor plants and flowers are subconscious symbols of life and vitality, and also enhance the energy of a room.

Having a symbol of aspiration or inspiration in the room again works on the unconscious mind to promote healing. If the person is religious, then an image to represent their belief system or an image of nature, where the individual has a continual view will assist in recovery and soothing the mind.

Playing soothing and gentle music also enhances the rate of healing, and should be incorporated with 'hands on' sessions to set an ambient mood.

Burning high quality incense or smudging a room to clear the negative energy discharged, is also of benefit.

(See chapter 10 on cleansing a room.)

Clothing and bedding also hold energy, so if a person has a fever and is sweating out toxins, they are literally lying in their own toxins. Changing clothing everyday and bedding every second day will clear excess build-up of lower vibrational energy.

THE ELEMENT OF WATER AND OUR PHYSICAL DIRECTION

Over 80% of our body is composed of the element water, and as we know, the moon affects the tides by its directional movement from the east to the west. In keeping with this concept, it makes sense to approach our spiritual practices, and even the direction in which we sleep, to flow with the cycles of the moon. Our internal waters are affected directly by this movement, so having your bed facing the axis of east/west will enhance balance. This is heightened with regards to an ill person who is trying to recover. When we face the northern direction, because our water is out of sync, it makes us tense; when we face the southern direction, it makes us weak. It is important to sleep with your head facing either the east or west axis. In this way we are staying in tune with the cycles of nature and the flow of universal energy.

EXERCISE

Many would consider exercise the last thing on their mind when they are ill; however, light exercise and being outside when the weather permits, is a vital element to health and wellness.

Participating in low-impact exercise such as brisk walking is generally best. It is important that the individual is sufficiently warm and does not overdo it. Choose when possible, to walk in nature. Simply being in a natural setting where the life force is abundant, tends to rub off on an ill individual and will enhance physical and mental well-being. A good routine is to walk for a comfortable time, then sit in meditation in a natural environment, and then walk again. This routine enhances balance and awareness. Engaging in other exercises that cultivate the enhancement of vital energy, such as Tai Chi or Chi Kung are also of great benefit, if you know how.

Another beneficial and pleasurable extension of this, is sexual intercourse. If the patient's strength permits, and the person is not suffering from any sexually transmitted or communicable diseases, then sexual congress should be allowed and even encouraged. The act of lovemaking is extremely beneficial in releasing the body's natural endorphins, and, thus, aids in the patients general mood, relaxation and well being. Contrary to many Taoist practices, this in no way weakens the life force of the patient, but rather increases the rate of healing and life force generated within the body, and is therefore beneficial in the healing process.

DIET, ALCOHOL, DRUGS AND HEALING

It makes sense to attend to a diet that is balanced with the five food groups with particular emphasis on fresh, organic and chi orientated foods. Fresh food is packed with life force that translates directly to you when you consume it. It should go without saying that recreational drugs and alcohol do not mix with illness. These substances directly affect the fragile life force of the sick person. At no time should a person who is ill use recreational drugs or alcohol as a form of escape. This does nothing for the advancement of healing in the body and the replenishment of vital energy. Of course, this does not mean that one should cease their prescribed medication from a General Practitioner. However if you are so inclined, giving Reiki to your medication before taking it, can enhance the positive qualities of the medicine.

KEEPING THE RIGHT COMPANY, A POSITIVE OUTLOOK

Keeping the right company when you are ill, is helpful in maintaining a positive outlook and the advancement of personal esteem and balance. The last thing you need when you are ill, is someone else telling you all about his/her problems, filling your mind with concerns and worry. It is a general rule to avoid people and situations that are filled with life-destroying and negative views. This has particular emphasis when someone is ill. The power of positive thinking has been well documented in relation to enhancing health and activating healing energies in the body. If you are confined to a bed with your illness, read or have someone read books to you which are inspirational and motivated toward a positive outlook. What we put into our bodies and mind, greatly influences our outlook and view of life.

In the words of the Buddha: *"We are what we think. All that we are arises with our thoughts. With our thoughts we make the world. Act or speak with an impure mind and trouble will follow you as the wheel follows the ox that draws the cart.*

We are what we think. All that we are arises with our thoughts. With our thoughts we make the world. Speak or act with a pure mind and happiness will follow you as your shadow, unshakable!"

INCORPORATING OTHER MODALITIES

Reiki is not the only form of alternative medicine out there, which can assist when we are out of balance. It is a good idea to incorporate other modalities which you feel may help your situation. Some other methods such as Chinese herbs, massage, shiatsu, acupuncture, naturopathy, reflexology, homeopathy, flower essence therapy and aromatherapy are all excellent approaches to healing and well being. However, be certain that the practitioner is fully trained and competent in their art, before investing your time, health and money. Combining Reiki with these modalities greatly enhances them in a variety of ways. For example, in most forms of bodywork and Shiatsu, practitioners have their hands in contact with the recipient's body most of the time. As Reiki is activated by touch, healing energy is being transmitted via the hands, directly into the meridians, organs, muscles and energy system of the individual. In homeopathy, aromatherapy and flower essence therapy, Reiki can enhance the positive healing qualities of the remedies by holding the medicine in your hands, and energizing them with the Reiki energy.

PREVENTIVE MEDICINE

The best approach to wellness is not to get sick in the first place, by paying attention to our physical bodies, our mental, and our emotional needs. Applying some of the preceding suggestions will certainly assist in this process. Good health is mostly common sense and listening to the wisdom of the body. Following these guidelines in conjunction with regular Reiki self-healing, enhances a positive outlook and creates balance physically, emotionally, mentally and spiritually in our lives. So many people are unhappy in their work, relationships and feel it is their lot in life to remain in an unsatisfying job for many years, to then retire and then expire. Following your dreams and passions are so important to living well and creating happiness. With continued use of Reiki for self-healing and by attending to some of the suggestions previously outlined, we can open the door to a better outlook for our health and our lives. Most importantly, do what you love to do.

REIKI FOR FIRST AID

First and foremost, Reiki is not designed to replace common sense and basic first aid procedures. However, Reiki is an excellent adjunct to first aid, and in most cases Reiki can be applied in conjunction with basic first aid. For example, if someone has cut himself, we can apply a bandage of some description, apply pressure to the wound, and at the same time, hold the area with our hands, transferring the Reiki energy. To be most affective in a first aid situation, it is suggested to start applying the

Reiki energy as soon as possible. The sooner we apply Reiki to the affected area, the sooner we are preventing unnecessary trauma setting in.

If it is not possible to place the hands in the affected area, we can use the law of correspondence.

Here we state that the part we are holding corresponds to the affected area, and imagine healing energy going to that place. At the Reiki I level, we simply place our hands wherever we can and state in our minds that the area we are touching now corresponds to the area in need. In addition to this, we can visualize this area beneath our hands as the affected area. Where possible we leave our hands in the area as long as possible. This may require you to be working on the area for a number of hours. Working in this way will greatly enhance the recovery and healing of the individual. It also makes a lot of sense to learn basic first aid. Courses are widely available, and are an essential adjunct to any practitioner of the healing arts.

PRACTICE AND SUPPORT

To further your relationship with Reiki, it is essential to put it into daily practice. Reiki works on the premise, like most things, that the more you put into it, the more you'll get back. So it makes sense to create the situations and time in your life to make this possible. What helps tremendously with practice is the support from like-minded friends on the path. At the AIRT we have regular get togethers, healing clinics and opportunities to review previous levels. This helps to strengthen and reconnect bonds made with old friends, to form new friendships and to practice with others who are interested in healing. As a result, many enduring relationships are born through Reiki.

If the teacher you learn from does not offer practice times or ongoing support after the workshop, then take a leap of faith and contact other teachers and practitioners to swap sessions. So often, the detriment of an individual's practice is due to the lack of support of like-minded people on the path. When we isolate ourselves, we potentially limit our growth.

Practical Practice

If a teaching or method has no practical application in your life, what use is it?

Engaging your mind with sensational phenomena may be entertaining for your mind but how does it contribute to healing? The following story illustrates this, and how one's practice should benefit not only yourself but others, in a practical and grounded way.

There is a story of an adept meditator in Buddha's time.

This man was a Sadhu or Holy man and through many years of practice had learnt to walk on water. One day, Buddha was walking along the river and met the Sadhu.

The Sadhu, not recognizing Buddha as an awakened being, tried to impress him with his magical abilities.

The Sadhu performed many magical feats, such as levitating, manifesting colourful energy fields, small objects and suchlike.

Each time he performed an act, the Buddha would respond

with enthusiasm, and would say: "That is amazing, what else can you do?"

Seeing that the Buddha was so impressed, the Sadhu saved his greatest act till last.

"I can walk across this river", he exclaimed, literally bursting with pride, and proceeded to walk on water. Buddha, seeing a boat nearby rowed the river and reached the other side. Once there he spoke to the Sadhu asking him how long it had taken him to accomplish this great feat. The Sadhu said filled with pride, "It took me thirty years!" Buddha said, "Wow!, thirty years to do that, it took me five minutes in that boat, what else can you do?"

At this point the Sadhu recognized the futility of his practice and became an avid follower of the Buddha's teachings. He then dedicated his life to the practical pursuit of awakening, grounded in the service and healing of all beings.

— Popular Buddhist fable, source unknown

So a teaching is of little worth if it does not liberate oneself or others. These days there are many vehicles to the spiritual path, so be sure the path you embark upon bears results. If we waste our time pursuing spiritual teachings that are shrouded in mystery, and blind belief, we are hardly developing self-reliance, compassion and healing. A spiritual teaching that teaches you to find your own awakening is a path worth pursuing. Buddha said, "I do not want anyone to follow me, I do not want to be your Guru, do not look at me, rather look at the teachings, try then for yourself and walk beside me, thou art the Buddha!"

REIKI I PRACTICE REQUIREMENTS

Having completed a Reiki I workshop, it is suggested to complete a self-healing session every day for a period of twenty one days, and complete at least twenty hands on sessions before considering Reiki II initiation. This is a suggested guide which if followed, will greatly enhance your understanding and integration of Reiki.

21 DAYS INTEGRATION

It is said that once having completed a Reiki I workshop, there is a three week period of integration which takes place. This is not really such a strange concept, when we consider that our entire energetic system has had a complete enhancement and realignment with the four initiations. During this time it is best to be aware of how the energy is shaping you. Many people report that they feel considerably different after a workshop and in the weeks that follow. Your personal experience is your own, and often we feel these changes in our emotional and mental selves. Common experiences range from a deeper sense of peace and serenity, inner calm and greater clarity. Many people report that once they have experienced the attunements in the workshop environment, the stresses of daily life don't seem to take hold or hold as much focus.

It is also suggested to nurture oneself during this period, and to pay attention to our bodies' needs.

One of the most effective ways to integrate the Reiki energy is to give yourself a daily self-treatment. Doing this greatly enhances your direct perception of the Reiki energy and allows the balancing of your physical, emotional, psychological and spiritual bodies. There are many benefits of daily practice. As we work on a daily level, we effectively build on previous sessions and as a result the degree of clearing, heightened sensitivity and one's perception becomes more emphasized. Sometimes strong emotions can arise as a result, of this type of intensive work. The important thing to remember is that it is all part of the healing process, and although it may not be very pleasant at the time, it is actually a good sign. Often, if this is occurring, it is the mind's ways of signalling some breakthrough of old dysfunctional patterns that we have held, on an energetic or an emotional level. It is best to continue self-healing especially when this is unfolding, as it will assist in the transition and healing taking place.

It is also good to have a friend or therapist to help if you are processing. Sometimes it can help a great deal when we talk about our problems with someone else, even if they just listen, that can be enough.

Keeping a Journal

Many people take up the suggestion of keeping a personal Reiki journal, to document their experiences and changes in themselves. Engaging in this process can be quite rewarding and act as a marker in times of transition. It may also simply off-load what's on your mind. Keeping a journal is a way to reflect on your personal growth and the changes that have occurred in your life as a result of your practice.

Requirements for a Traditional Reiki I Workshop

Each teacher of Reiki brings his own unique teaching style and approach when passing on his understanding. People are so varied, it is essential to have a variety of teachers to express in a way that speaks to other like-minded people. With this in mind, there is a certain content one should cover within a Reiki I workshop, and it goes as follows:

1. Four Reiki I Initiations. Two each day, either morning and afternoon or one each day over four consecutive days.
2. Students are shown traditional hand positions, and have the opportunity to practice at least two full one hour sessions within the workshop environment.
3. Students have an opportunity to explore intuitive approaches to hands on healing.
4. Students are shown the application of centering procedures, personal boundaries and related practices.
5. Students are instructed on the oral Reiki History, the importance of lineage and where they fit into the Reiki Lineage.
6. Explanation of initiations and why they are an important part of the Reiki System.
7. Practice requirements are given during and after the workshop.
8. Students receive a manual of procedures and information on Reiki and its variety of applications.

9. Students receive a copy of the Reiki Principles and a Certificate in First Degree Reiki upon completion.
10. Total Workshop duration: 14 Hours.

Chapter 9

'For the things we have to learn, before we can learn them, we learn by doing them.'

— ***Aristotle***

FREQUENTLY ASKED QUESTIONS

Q: *What makes the Reiki System unique from other healing modalities?*

A: Reiki is one of the few energy healing systems that do not require focused intent or specific mental imagery to create positive results. When you think of all the healing energy streams around these days, one could use the analogy of our hand. The palm of our hand represents the source of all things and our fingers are these various forms of energy work. One finger is Reiki, another is Chi Kung, and another is Prana and so on. They all come from the same source, yet each one has its unique expression, form and style. Another unique feature of this system is the source of the healing energy. Reiki does not come from one's own energy field. It is simply a by-product of the interaction with the Universal healing frequency, and the individual's energy system. In a nutshell, the system requires a passive and non-doing approach. It is not only a healing tool for another, but also works well for one's personal healing.

Q: *What do I think of when I'm doing Reiki; do I need to act in a certain way?*

A: At the Reiki I level, we simply observe what we are sensing and that is all. With the higher Reiki levels there is a greater emphasis on mental imagery, however, at this level, we are generally trying to get our heads out of the way to develop stillness while we facilitate the transference of Universal energy. Once the alignments are in order (Reiki Attunements), the healing energy is activated by touch, and this is why it is not necessary to concentrate.

In the words of Mrs Takata: " Hands on – Reiki on, Hands off – Reiki off!"

Q: *Is it necessary to visualize anything whilst facilitating Reiki?*

A: At the Reiki I level, it is not a requirement to visualize anything to make it happen.

As previously mentioned, the Reiki energy flows once the hands are within the energy field or on the body of the recipient. In the Reiki levels beyond first degree, visualization can be incorporated into your session. This is achieved by visualizing symbols in the body, to direct the Reiki energy for specific situations. Some practitioners like to visualize themselves as empty vessels for the energy to pass through or may visualize the energy going to a particular part of the body of the recipient, however this is not essential as the energy is doing this by itself. These visualizations can assist as a means of focus for your own mind, by keeping attention and awareness on the task at hand. Just remember that it is the Divine Intelligence of Reiki doing the healing and not yourself.

Q: *Are abilities like clairvoyance, psychic ability and seeing auras a necessary part of Reiki?*

A: These sorts of phenomena are not essential to facilitate an effective Reiki session. The tools that are imparted in the attunement process, awaken the stream of Universal healing energy from yourself to the recipient. With practice, some of these inner abilities naturally begin to unfold. Each person tends to develop these abilities at a different rate, and it is largely dependant upon how much one practices and applies the methods taught at the various Reiki levels. Certainly, specific attunements in the levels also focus on the opening of the inner senses. So, it is a balance between your own inner unfolding which comes through practice, and the attunements that open specific doorways of energy within the being on a clairvoyant level. Don't be too concerned if you are or are not experiencing these sorts of phenomena. If you are, then that's okay and if not, then that is also okay. Reiki does not require any special talent or spiritual predisposition to achieve positive results.

Q: *Once you have completed Reiki I, can you lose the healing energy or can it be taken away by a negative experience?*

A: Provided the recipient has received the four initiations in Reiki I by a qualified teacher, the energy stays with the individual for the rest of his life. It can never be lost or hindered once the person has received these alignments. Having received the Reiki attunements, instils a protective quality within the being, and by simply facilitating Reiki, this protective quality manifests.

Q: *Is there anyone who does Reiki I and it doesn't work?*

A: The Reiki initiations are a specific formula, which have a specific result. This result creates a pathway for transmitting the Reiki energy. This alignment always occurs, regardless of whether your personal belief is uncertain. It makes no difference if you believe in your ability. Simply, if you have an energetic system, which everyone does, then you have what it takes to become a channel for Reiki energy.

Q: *If you are giving yourself Reiki and fall asleep, does the energy switch off?*

A: Reiki energy is not dependant on your state of consciousness. If the Reiki energy works without your thoughts and is activated by touch, then no matter where your state of consciousness, the healing will still take place. I have personally experienced this when I was receiving Reiki from one of my teachers and he fell asleep whilst giving me Reiki. As he was snoring in my ear, which was quite amusing and disturbing, the Reiki energy was still flowing strongly through his hands. Quite an unusual way to prove it for myself. So the good news is, you can get quite a lot of self-healing done when you are asleep.

Q: *Are some people better at Reiki than others?*

A: Some people have a natural pre-disposition to the healing ability and may be more attuned to subtle energies. However, even if you don't naturally have this ability, you also will develop it once initiated. This sensitivity is also cultivated through on-going practice, some people just develop this faster than others.

Q: *Are all the Reiki systems out there the same?*

A: No, not all Reiki systems offered are the same.

Many people have put their own ideas into Reiki and have changed the original system and symbols to suit their needs. Further to this, many teachers have not informed their students of the changes made. The result of this often leads to distorted views and misunderstanding of what the original system contains. As a result, the passing of information and techniques does vary greatly from teacher to teacher. Naturally, each teacher brings their unique style to the Reiki system. Where the danger lies is in the changing, removal or additions to the symbols or initiations, which are essentially the foundation of the Reiki system. Some of the confusion regarding the different systems currently available, stem from the teacher concerned being improperly trained from the outset. Unfortunately, all the best intentions in the world are not enough. If we don't have the correct procedures for making the alignment with the Reiki energy, it simply won't work to its full potential. So it is important to receive the right transmission, methodology and teachings in order to achieve the best results.

Q: *Can Reiki Harm instead of heal?*

A: The Reiki energy is one of the highest and most gentle forms of Universal power available to mankind at this point in history. In itself, the energy is always safe and will only go to the places in the being that requires healing. This is always for the highest good of the beings concerned. Where Reiki is not safe, is when people combine the original system with other esoteric practices, which may be in themselves dualistic in nature. So it depends upon how it is used.

Q: *What is meant by dualistic energy?*

A: Dualistic energy and practices do not operate solely from the source of Universal energy. Examples of these would be Chi energy work, which can be used for healing, or in the case of some martial arts which can be used to deliver a destructive blow to the body. It depends upon how it is used. For example, a martial arts expert can use the Chi energy to break a bone through a single blow or the energy can be used to heal a physical alignment. It depends upon the focus and intent of the person facilitating the energy. Reiki on the other hand can only be used to promote healing, it is always safe, gentle and is a passive form of energy work.

Crystals are another example of dualistic energy. Many people assume that all crystals are good and do specific things for you. Crystals are dualistic in nature, which means it depends upon how they are used and how they have been used in the past. Crystals are basically amplifiers.

If you are angry and hold a crystal as a quick fix for the anger, all that occurs is the crystal amplifies your anger, unless your belief is so strong that your intention creates a placebo effect. An un-programmed crystal is neutral or dualistic.

Now if a crystal is programmed with healing energy or a positive vibration for example, then it can be used for healing. In order for the crystal to be used in this way, it should be cleansed of any previous programming. So, we can see that one needs to be very careful, even when dabbling with innocent looking crystals.

(For more information on crystals and healing, see chapter 13.)

Q: *Is Reiki a Cult or Religion?*

A: Reiki is neither a Cult or a Religion. The system certainly derives its base from Buddhist traditions, which in themselves are philosophical and psychologically based. The Reiki system known in the West is not based on an individual dogma or structured belief system. It is however, a spiritual system, which is experientially based and contains principles for gaining self-empowerment and personal unfoldment. There are certain branches of the original system which require the individual to take refuge in certain Buddhist practices and ideas. Western Reiki, which was derived from Hawayo Takata's teaching, is more broad based focusing on general spirituality with nondenominational views.

Q: *Does Reiki work every time?*

A: There is always some benefit in receiving a Reiki session; the degree of what is healed varies from person to person. Some results can be life changing or in the miraculous category, and at other times it is an on-going and gradual process. Certainly there are immediate benefits, such as relaxation and reduced stress. It also has provided immediate relief for a variety of aches and pains.

Q: *What is Absent healing?*

A: Absent healing is the ability to send healing energy at a distance. This method is taught in Level II. With this ability we can assist in the positive outcomes of situations of the past, present or future. We can also heal others at a distance as well as heal various emotional issues.

Q: *How long does it take to become a practitioner of Reiki?*

A: Generally, one becomes a Practitioner of Reiki after one has received the four attunements of Reiki I. Most people who wish to start a Reiki practice, however, usually complete Reiki level II.

This is usually completed after three to six months of practice, then one may practice in the conventional sense. The emphasis is always on experience, a good understanding and personal integration.

Q: *If Reiki is from the Universe and we are a part of this, why can't everyone just do it at will?*

A: The problem we face is that we have forgotten the way. Let us use the analogy of our own energy system as an antenna, and Reiki as a frequency we are trying to pick up. It is not enough to just will it on. It's as if we are missing the dials to tune the energy. There is a specific way to awaken or tune in this ability. If you don't have the method, or empowerment for that matter, it just won't happen. Many people assume that all forms of healing ability are Reiki energy. People often comment, 'Oh, I do Reiki' and yet they have not received any of the attunements in the tradition.

Now, this is not to negate other healing systems out there, they are equally valid; the point is that there are many different methods of channelling healing energy. The Reiki system on its own is quite unique. Many people come to Reiki from previous experiences of having had something happen. They have some healing ability, yet it wasn't on call whenever they needed it, a bit hit and miss, if you like. The general consensus is, that once they received the attunements it was no longer hit and miss, it worked all the time, every time. In other words, no static in the antenna.

Chapter 10

'The purpose of life is not to be happy – but to matter, to be productive, to be useful, to have it make some difference that you lived at all.'

— Leo Rosten

REIKI II

Reiki II or Second degree is the next step in the traditional Western Reiki System.

Reiki II is a further increase of one's capacity to work with Universal energy, and opens the door to increased personal growth and empowerment. In Second degree Reiki, participants receive the first three sacred symbols of this level. These are learnt as a means of performing absent healing and working on many new and creative ways with the Reiki energy.

In Reiki II there is also an increased empowerment with the Second degree initiation.

What the Reiki II Initiation Achieves

The Reiki II initiation requires the four Reiki I initiations to work effectively. For example, if someone has completed Reiki I with another teacher and wanted to participate in a Reiki II workshop, they would need to be re-initiated into the particular Reiki lineage of the new teacher with the four Reiki I initiations. Without this, the Reiki II initiation will not work to its fullest capacity. The primary reason for this, is that each initiation works in succession from each previous one. If one teacher's initiation procedure differs from that of another, then the bestowal of a new level loses its continuity, and therefore, the empowerment is incomplete.

As a result, the student will not be fully aligned with the particular lineage of the new initiating teacher. It is for this reason that the Reiki II initiation requires the previous attunements given in sequence for them to be activated within the student.

The Reiki II initiation expands on the pathway created by the four Reiki I initiations. It highlights the Sacral Chakra on a general level, and expands one's capacity to channel Universal energy. In particular, this initiation gives the empowerment of the three Reiki II symbols. These empowerments are activated through the palm chakras.

This initiation doubles the capacity to channel Reiki energy, by expanding the channel at the Crown, Heart, and Palm Chakras.

Things to Consider Before Learning Reiki II

Before taking the next step in the Reiki system, one should consider one's motivation for advancing a level. One should also consider one's level of understanding and experience in the practices of Reiki I. It is generally suggested that a student should actively use Reiki I, for approximately three months. Naturally, one may wish to do this sooner or later depending upon one's predisposition to the healing arts, their previous experience and personal preferences.

WHAT ARE BOOSTER INITIATIONS?

The Reiki Booster initiations are present in all the AIRT Reiki levels. These initiations hold the basic framework for the specific alignments of each level, and act as a way to boost the practitioners' level of power. The Booster attunements also act as a blessing, and a way to enjoy the experience that one receives from the attunement procedures. The Booster initiations are not an essential part of the empowerment procedures, and one does not need to be reliant on receiving Booster attunements. However, Booster attunements are very powerful and are a way to generate a large amount of spiritual power and energy in someone who receives them.

These attunements can be facilitated by practitioners who are not teachers of Reiki, provided they have completed and received the initiations of level 3A. At this level the student can facilitate the Reiki level I Booster and the Reiki level II Booster attunements. The Reiki II Booster attunement should only be given to a Reiki practitioner who has completed and received the Reiki II initiation from a qualified Reiki instructor of the same lineage. The Reiki I Booster on the other hand, can be given to anyone who wishes to experience the Reiki energy on a personal level. This particular attunement empowers an individual with the Reiki energy, however this alignment is temporary. One requires the four Reiki I attunements in sequence by a qualified teacher, to have a permanent Reiki alignment.

THE REIKI SYMBOLS

The Reiki symbols act as pathways to the Reiki energy and enable the student to direct healing energy in specific ways.

In recent years, many teachers who were taught by Hawayo Takata have been sharing information on the symbols and their uses. In addition to this there has been an explosion of information published in books and in particular over the internet, on Reiki symbols, initiation procedures, etc.

One of the Reiki taboos as taught by teachers of the old western schools, is the publishing of the Reiki symbols. There are many pros and cons to this argument. Firstly, in publishing sacred material there is always the chance that people, human nature being what it is, will misuse this power.

What is often misunderstood, is that this knowledge is of no use without the actual empowerments from a qualified Reiki teacher. Without these empowerments, performing these procedures is like trying to drive a car without any keys – it simply won't work.

However on the flip side of this, is the sharing of information and the education for practitioners who may or may not have accurate depictions of the Reiki symbols. In viewing these symbols the student can at least know what they have by comparison and, thus, correct their techniques, if need be.

In the old Reiki schools in the West, it was common practice in a Reiki II workshop that having viewed the Reiki symbols, one would need to commit them to memory and then burn them at the end of the workshop. Unfortunately, this practice, largely results in a great deal of Reiki practitioners not being able to remember the Reiki symbols, or having completely inaccurate depictions from the originals.

Today, most Reiki teachers have moved on from this practice and now supply their Reiki II students with visual representations of the Reiki symbols for personal reference.

With all this in mind, I have decided to publish the original Reiki symbols that were written in Takata's handwriting. As far as Western Universal Reiki goes, these are as close to the source of Takata's teachings and the system that Dr. Usui taught to his non-Buddhist students. The sharing of these symbols is hoped to assist in the understanding of information amongst practitioners, and to open the door to greater freedom in the methods expressed in Universal Reiki.

(To see Mrs Takata's original Reiki symbols see chapter 18.)

THE INTEGRATION OF BODY, SPEECH AND MIND

The Reiki symbols are, in effect, living energy fields. Each time a symbol is drawn, the frequency of that symbol manifests. It is vitally important if we are to obtain the highest potential of this energy field, that these symbols are drawn and pronounced precisely. In some Reiki schools, teachers advocate that it is the mantra that holds the power, while in other schools a teacher may advocate that it is the symbol that holds the power. In actuality, the mantra and the symbols themselves are equal components to a third energy being manifested, which is a result of the two parts combined.

In the Reiki system, a symbol represents the Body element, and the Mantra that goes with the symbol represents the speech element. These two combined create the element of mind or the actualization of the symbol's energy summoned. It is essential to summon both energies in this practice, as this creates the third element or totality of the symbol's energy. For example, if we only state the symbol and not draw or visualize the symbol, then we have only one element and are missing its other essential components.

At the beginner's stage, it is essential to practice these forms on a regular basis, one should know these forms and be able to sign these without relying on memory.

Once a student has embodied these symbols on an inner level, these three elements come together without effort.

It is when one signs these symbols without conscious effort, that one has gone beyond concept and form and has realized the true nature of the Reiki symbols.

THE REIKI II SYMBOLS

We will now look at each of the three Reiki symbols presented in the second degree class.

The words are in Japanese, although their meaning in a modern Japanese dictionary is not necessarily literal. The language used comes from ancient origins, and throughout time the meaning in context to the symbol has evolved as the system has passed through a variety of cultures.

Cho Ku Rei

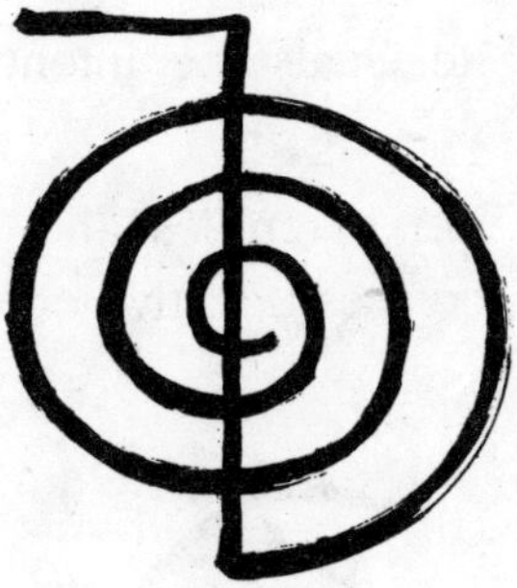

Cho Ku Rei

The first symbol is known as the 'Power symbol' and is spoken amongst the Reiki initiated with the symbol's Mantra: CHO KU REI.

This mantra was given to the symbols as it was passed throughout the tradition.

The first symbol traditionally taught is the CHO KU REI.

Cho Ku Rei (pronounced cho koo ray)

This symbol's uses are:

- This symbol activates the Reiki energy. It draws 100% of the Reiki energy to one point fully focused.
- This symbol empowers all the other symbols and is usually used at the end of a sequence of symbols.

- Envisioned in three dimensions it can be used to draw energy from the field, and in the opposite fashion to draw energy into a point on the body.
- Cho Ku Rei can be drawn over the hands before commencing a Reiki session which activates the Reiki energy immediately in the hands.
- Drawn or infused through the crown chakra this symbol will energize when the energy field is depleted.
- The Cho Ku Rei seals the intent for a healing or affirmation.
- The Cho Ku Rei magnifies and increases positive energy and decreases negative energy.

Sei He Ki

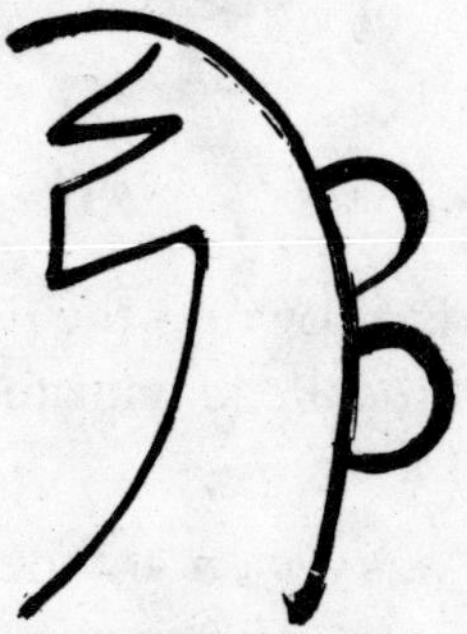

Sei He Ki

The second symbol taught traditionally is the SEI HE KI, also described as the "mental symbol".

Sei He Ki (pronounced say hay key)

This symbol's uses are:

- Sei He Ki establishes Personal Boundaries, and acts as a filter to lesser emotional/mental states.

- This symbol acts as a way to seal the Thymus Chakra and protects an individual from lower vibrational energy, psychic influences and negativity.
- This symbol activates the Divine Intelligence within, activating the highest good within a situation or in a person. Creating order where there is disharmony.
- Sei He Ki is the key to accessing the 'Transpersonal Self', internal dialogue and clairvoyant information.
- Used alone or in conjunction with other symbols, it serves as protection from lower vibration energy.

Hon Sha Ze Sho Nen

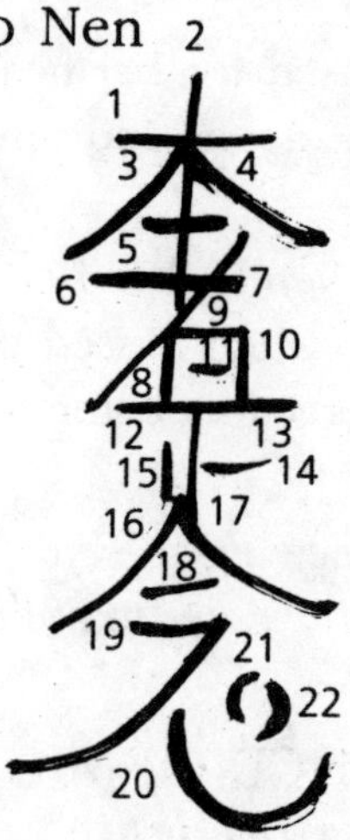

Hon Sha Ze Sho Nen

The third symbol taught at Reiki II is the HON SHA ZE SHO NEN, this symbol is also referred to as the "bridge symbol".

Hon Sha Ze Sho Nen (pronounced hon shar zay show nen)

This symbol's uses are:

- The Hon Sha Ze Sho Nen is used to transcend time and space. It enables a bridging of energy and symbols from one place to another, regardless of time or distance. Energy can be sent whether it is past, present or projecting healing energy to the future. In effect this symbol acts as a bridge.
- Hon Sha Ze Sho Nen enables the practitioner to direct energy and symbols to more than one place at once. It also bridges energy flow from one point of the body to another, especially where the hands are not in contact.
- This symbol is used for balancing the chakras and working into the organs and inner structures of the body.
- Hon Sha Ze Sho Nen is also used for centering in the present moment, when passed through the body in the preliminary practices before commencing a Reiki II session.
- Used in absent healing to send healing energy and symbols to specific issues to affect current situations.

THE IMPORTANCE OF SIGNING THE REIKI SYMBOLS

In learning the Reiki symbols we not only want to commit these to memory, we want to work with them on a deep and ever evolving level. In Reiki II we draw the symbols many times over, aiming for perfection and full awareness every time. Each time we sign a Reiki symbol we are signing the name of the sacred. In doing so we honour the divinity of the universal energy and we honour ourselves. Again, it comes down to right motivation. If we take a lazy and unconscious approach to signing the symbols, we are affirming this in ourselves. So always aim for excellence. Much like the Zen practice of signing one Japanese Kanji, thousands upon thousands of times to perfect the form. If we make a mistake, when signing a symbol, we sign a Cho Ku Rei over the symbol and start again. At the AIRT students draw the Reiki symbols many hundreds of times within a workshop to instil the essence of each symbol. With time a deeper language begins to form in the symbols, and the Wisdom of Reiki begins to permeate. When the symbol signs you, then you are at the beginning of a new level of understanding.

NON-TRADITIONAL REIKI SYMBOLS

Non-traditional Reiki symbols are becoming more and more popular in Reiki classes worldwide. It is important to note here, that if a 'non-traditional' Reiki symbol is taught, it should be done clearly, so as not to create confusion within the Reiki system. Unfortunately, many Reiki teachers do not make this distinction, and many students work with additional symbols rather than the ones described previously for Reiki II.

Teaching symbols which differ from the three traditional Reiki symbols clearly show a deviation from the original Reiki system. As stated previously, one also requires initiation or an empowerment to use a particular symbol, and this needs to be bestowed by someone who is empowered to give such a transmission. This is not to say that other symbols do not hold power, however, it is paramount that a teacher giving a symbol be empowered to give it appropriately, with the correct empowerment and permission necessary to make this alignment in the student. A student should seek this information from a teacher when considering the second level of Reiki.

It is important to know what you will be covering throughout the workshop, that the symbols taught have lineage and the teacher concerned is empowered to pass these on appropriately.

MODES OF PERCEPTION

The symbols of the traditional Reiki II level offer the student a number of new resources in working hands on, as well as in Absent Healing. These symbols, directed with specific intent will enhance energy flow and direction of the Universal energy, thus, enabling further abilities as a practitioner.

At this level we can utilize the Reiki symbols to establish our personal boundaries, clear any blockages or lower energetic patterns, balance the energy centres and access information from a variety of means on visual, auditory and kinaesthetic levels.

PERCEPTION

As human beings the way in which we take on information from our outer and inner worlds operates from our perception. The most common way that we can utilize these methods is through our Visual, Kinaesthetic and

Auditory abilities. On a daily level we constantly operate out of these modes of perception. When we see a nice looking car for example, we see the image visually. This may elicit an emotion or feeling as we visualize ourselves driving the car, and our internal dialogue may be along the lines of " I'd love to own one of those". So, just in that moment we may have operated unconsciously on a visual level (seeing the car and using the imagination); on a kinaesthetic level (feeling associated to the car, psychosomatic responses to the car), and lastly auditory (the internal dialogue associated with our response to the car and our observations).

Our modes of perception operate constantly, without our conscious awareness of their presence. Intuitively, our modes of perception are very useful in healing work and can be used to greatly assist in the fine tuning of our sessions. These benefits also filter out into our daily lives with regard to accessing information, decision-making and living more intuitively.

By using our perception as a tool to access information, we are simply slowing down our usual processes. By asking the right kind of questions inwardly, we can access information with awareness of what arises on a conscious level. Everyone has this ability; all we need to do is know how to perceive it.

ACCESSING OUR CURRENT STATE

Also described as 'checking in', this is a preliminary procedure used before we begin our hands on session. This technique is also a way to monitor or access information that bypasses our physical mind and goes directly to our higher or our Transpersonal Self.

In a way it is much like using an internal pendulum to access 'yes' and 'no' responses, and basic replies to simple questions.

This approach works best when we are precise and direct with our inquiry.

Procedure:

Place your hands on your upper chest and ask the question in your mind: "Am I energetically clear to commence this healing session?"

Upon asking this question, there is often an immediate response. This occurs through one of our modes of perception, primarily: Visual, Auditory or Kinaesthetic.

The following are examples which indicate a 'Yes' response.

Visual	-	seeing a bright colour or positive imagery.
Kinaesthetic	-	feeling a rising feeling in the upper chest or head, or an engaging and embracing feeling.
Auditory	-	the word in our head 'Yes' or some other dialogue to this effect.

A 'No' response could be:

Visual	-	Seeing or sensing a dull colour or experiencing negative imagery.
Kinaesthetic	-	A sinking feeling in the lower belly or pushing back, pulling away feeling.

Auditory - The word 'No' or words to this effect.

These are common examples, although they are not exclusive in their interpretation. Through working with awareness and perception, a pattern for receiving information tends to unfold. As this evolves, we start to see a pattern of what modes we commonly operate from. These are the ways of seeing beyond our ordinary state of perception.

When asking a question on this level, the response is almost always immediate. So it is best to go with your first response. Many of us are taught from an early age not to trust our intuitive responses, and to look for a logical and cognitive understanding. So when someone asks a question of themselves, the first obstacle we encounter is our ego mind, in the form of Doubt, Judgment and Fear.

Here is an example to illustrate the point of internal doubt we can encounter when doing this for the first time.

"Am I energetically clear? Yes! No, of course you're not, that's why you are here, because you have so many problems. What makes me think I can do this?, I've never been able to do these type of things", etc. You get the picture. So the response was "Yes" to the question, then the conditioned mind, stepped in to put you straight.

The response was Auditory in nature, with a little self doubt thrown in, followed by a side order of Self-Judgment. This is relatively common in beginning to trust our inner voice; it takes time to override these types of conditioning. The good news is, with practice and persistence, it does become easier. The key thing to look for is the first response, whether it be visual, auditory or kinaesthetic.

This same procedure can be applied to just about any decision or choice to be made. Using this technique, we bypass our physical mind and go directly to our intuition (inner knowing). Another extension of this is to hold an object with awareness.

For example: You may want to purchase a book. Hold the book in your hands and tune in. Ask the question: "Is this an appropriate book for me now?", and wait for your immediate response. Try it and see for yourself! This is your intuition talking.

Another excellent way to access your intuitive responses is using the Bai Hui point, which is situated on the crown of our heads. To find this exact point, one draws a line from the bottom of the lobe to the top of the ear, and follow this angle up to the top of the head. Another way to find this point is to place your own hands on your head and measure, eight finger widths from your original hairline, back to the centre of your head.

This point is a major point of energy flow and is a direct way to gain an intuitive response. In the same situation as illustrated before, one could place an object on their Bai Hui point and tune in for a response on a visual, kinaesthetic or auditory level.

TRANSFERENCE

The term transference describes the taking on of another's symptoms as a result of a healing session. These symptoms can occur in a variety of ways either physically, emotionally, psychically and/or spiritually. Often the reason for this occurring is due to the neglect of establishing appropriate personal boundaries before commencing a session. It is vitally important to have an awareness of boundaries whenever an exchange occurs. The benefit of working with the Reiki energy is that the very nature of Reiki has a strong protective quality. This protection is imparted during the initiation procedures. As a result, whenever we facilitate healing for another, this protective quality of the healing energy is always with us. Above and beyond this, we can greatly enhance our boundaries by engaging in the 'Protection and Boundaries' procedures described in the following pages. When we look at most traditional forms of hands on healing, whether it be from the ancient Shamanic indigenous traditions or Western mysticism, there is always some preliminary procedure that a practitioner follows, to either call in one's allies or the correct forces to assist in a healing outcome. Therefore, it makes sense to apply this fundamental law to our healing work. This becomes more emphasized when we are dealing with very ill or negative people. When we establish our intent for healing and set up the appropriate conditions, we greatly enhance our personal and spiritual strength. The following is a procedure for activating your personal boundaries with the second Reiki II symbol, the SEI HE KI.

ESTABLISHING PERSONAL BOUNDARIES

This is an invaluable practice for anyone in health care professions, i.e., nursing, hospice, mental health, or in general for times when we feel that we are taking on unnecessary emotional or mental energy from another.

The nature of Reiki has a protective quality that is present once a person has received the four alignments from Reiki I. However, there are certain situations that call for additional protection. The Sei He Ki is a direct way to boost our psychic defences when applied to our thymus chakra. Many of us would have experienced being in the presence of someone who is depressed or sad. After a period of being exposed to this energy, it starts to rub off on us and we begin to feel heavy or down ourselves. This is a classic example of transference.

Transference can occur in a number of ways, and in particular during hands on work.

A regular comment from remedial massage therapists is that they often experience pain in their hands in relation to a tension spot on their client, or experience the feeling of being drained, after a session.

Another example is when someone is conducting a session and experiences the clients' symptoms in his or her own body. This is referred to as "telesomatic transference".

Some native healers use this method for diagnosing and removing harmful influences in their clients. However they are specialists, and often have preliminarily processes which they engage in to deal with this energy in an appropriate way.

In the Reiki system, there are ways to establish the appropriate boundaries. As a precaution to transference occurring, we use the protective quality of the Sei He Ki in conjunction with our Thymus Chakra, (the thymus being the seat of our immune system). The thymus is located, one inch below the meeting points of our collarbones in the upper chest.

Procedure:

Place one hand over the Thymus Chakra and one hand on the back of the neck where the neck and shoulders meet. This point is the vertebra that is protruding slightly beyond the others, and is referred to as C7 in massage. Now visualize a Sei He Ki in the colour sky blue, under both your hands.

Visualizing the colour blue is a visual tool to focus the mind and is also a colour metaphysically associated with protection and higher energies. If you are having a block with visualizing, just sense it or state the fact in your mind; the effect is much the same.

Having sealed your boundaries, this effectively establishes this state energetically for the duration of the healing session. This process is also repeated at the completion of the session, in order to disconnect from the client. The procedure is the same.

This exercise can also be extended into daily life. When we are in a public place, for example a hospital, it is not always possible to drop everything and place our hands back and front on our Thymus Chakra, especially if we have an on-looking audience. So this can be facilitated as a visualization or intention. Further to this, we can imagine the Sei He Ki wrapped around us with one part of the symbol on either side of our body in the colour blue, much like wearing a protective coat or cape around you.

CLEARING ENERGY

Now, there are times when we do take on the process of another in the form of transference. When this does occur, we can clear this lower vibration energy from ourselves by passing the Sei He Ki through our energy field, thereby raising the body's frequency. When we do this, the lower frequency is transmuted by the higher vibration of the Reiki symbol. We can also clear ourselves when we are feeling sluggish or when our own personal vibration is low. Remember, the Reiki symbols are living energy fields. Each time a symbol is drawn, the field effect occurs.

Effectively, by doing this we raise our vibration and, thus, strengthen our energy field.

Procedure:

Visualize or draw a large Sei He Ki in front of you, seeing it in the colour blue. The symbol should be the same size as you, and directly in front. Now in your mind's eye, pass this symbol through your energy field and body, back and forth three times. When we do this, we raise our vibration and resonance to a higher frequency and the lower vibration energy is transmuted to this level. To expand on this, we can also affirm in our minds the following: "I now clear any lesser or lower energies, these energies now leave this vessel and all lower energy is now transformed into the highest good."

This whole process may be repeated three times or until you feel clear.

OTHER METHODS OF CLEANSING

Some other ways to cleanse yourself energetically, is to burn native herbs and use the smoke to cleanse or 'smudge' your energy field. Smudging is an ancient practice of using particular herbs to ceremonially cleanse the body and energy field of negative influences and feelings. These herbs have a direct effect on the human energy field, and promote energetic clarity.

Herbs that are commonly used for cleansing are sage, cedar, sweet grass and sandalwood.

Smudge sticks are widely available in most New Age stores.

Salt water

Salt water is another excellent gift from nature that cleanses the human energy field almost immediately. A swim in the ocean for 5 to 10 minutes, will clear any lower energy from your field and restore balance to your field. If the ocean is not accessible, a salt bath is another good alternative.

Place two generous handfuls of rock salt or sea salt into a bath, and raise the water to a comfortable depth and temperature. Soak for 15 minutes and allow the salt to melt away any lower vibration energy.

Cleansing Breaths Procedure

When you are just about ready to get out of the bath, release the water and focus on your 'out breaths'. As you are breathing out, visualize that any remaining discursive thoughts, feelings or energy is leaving your body with the water, and that this energy is leaving via the palms of your hands and the soles of your feet. You will generally feel relaxed but a little drained from this process.

Once finished, have a quick shower to wash off the salt, lay down and apply a self-healing procedure for about 15 minutes. This will revitalize your energy field.

During the self-healing, focus on your 'in breath', this will also enhance the re-energizing process.

The process of releasing the breath can be used anytime to centre and remove unwanted energy. If you are standing or seated, imagine the breath leaving via the soles of the feet and going into the earth, where the natural forces of nature can transmute this energy.

CLEANSING ROOMS OR A LOCATION WITH THE REIKI SYMBOLS

It makes sense to do a spring clean every now and then, but how often do we consider our energetic environment? Have you ever entered a room and got the 'heebie-jeebies', or just felt like you wanted to leave because it didn't feel right? This is often the result of lower vibrational energy within a room.

There is a simple procedure to clear these lower vibrations and to call in a higher frequency.

If you operate your sessions out of a room on a regular basis, then this practice can be a regular event and will enhance your personal environment.

Places of illness and death are lower vibration energy magnets. Funeral directors, hospitals, veterinary clinics, etc. This procedure can also be sent as an absent healing procedure.

Clearing Rooms Procedure

Firstly, open a window or door, this allows the old energy to disperse.

We begin in the centre of the room.

We centre ourselves and seal our personal boundaries as described previously. Once we feel centred, we go to a corner of the room. With one hand on our heart and the other hand extended in front of us, we sign a large Sei He Ki in the air. This can be drawn with our hand or we can incorporate a smudge stick or incense stick into the procedure by signing the symbol with the stick.

Now we walk to the next corner and whilst we are walking, we affirm either silently or aloud, "I now clear any lesser or lower energies from this room, all is transformed into the highest good." Having arrived at the next corner, we then sign another large Sei He Ki and repeat the affirmation to the next corner and so on, until we have reached the corner where we started.

BRINGING HEALING POWER INTO A ROOM

This procedure follows the clearing procedure.

Having cleared the room, we can now bring in a positive influence.

1. Stand at the centre of the room and face east.

   Holding your hand in front of you, sign a large Cho Ku Rei to that direction, stating the name of the symbol three times. Now bring your hand to your heart centre and cup the symbol here also.

2. Face north and sign the symbol again, bringing your hand back to your cupped hand at the heart.

   Now you have two cupped symbols at your heart.

3. Face west and repeat the process, one to the west, one cupped at your heart.

4. Repeat the same for the south.

5. Face east again (you should have four symbols cupped in your hand now).

   Draw Cho Ku Rei again over your cupped hand, followed by:

   Hon Sha Ze Sho Nen, Sei He Ki and Cho Ku Rei.

6. Give a prayer of intent.

7. Now as if you have a ball in your hands, throw this energy up into the sky.

   Leave your hands out to the sides, you will often feel the energy raining down over you and into the room.

This exercise will call the Reiki energy into the room. You may wish to use one of the other symbols for each direction or a symbol stack, see which symbol feels appropriate for each situation.

These procedures act as a powerful way to not only clear lower resonance energy, but to evoke the Reiki energy as well.

If we follow the Universal law that love and fear

cannot occupy the same space, then when we establish the Reiki energy in a room like this on a regular basis, we build up the higher frequency of love. This also has a protective quality; in a way we are building a sanctuary of love and positivity. It is a type of 'spiritual teflon coating'; negativity just slides off and can't penetrate the positive energy field.

These procedures also work especially well in absent healing. I know of a teacher who sent absent healing to his classroom each morning using this technique, and was astounded by the ways in which his students behaved. He also noticed that when he didn't, how much they did misbehave and caused trouble. So when we facilitate this procedure, we are offering a positive energy field that will benefit all concerned.

PURIFICATION

We can actively cleanse ourselves with Reiki, when used in a particular way. This aids in removing obstacles to our path and healing.

The procedure is as follows:

1. Sit or lie in a room, close your eyes and bring to mind a particular problem, emotion, illness, etc. Think about this and make this issue strong in your mind.
2. Now focusing on this issue, ask yourself the question: 'If this issue resided in my body, where would it reside?' Now tune into your body and locate the root cause of this issue.
3. Place your hands on this area and give yourself self-healing.

4. Now think to yourself, 'If this issue had a form, sensation or colour what would it be?' Imagine this issue in a particular form, colour or sensation.
5. **Place your hands** on this part of your body and imagine a brilliant white light penetrating this issue, reducing it in size, dissolving or extracting this from your body. Keep doing this until there is no remnant of this issue left.
6. Once this issue has been removed and purified, imagine a sphere or some symbol that holds power and spiritual meaning for you. See the symbol in this place, radiating light, healing and protection. This can be imagined throughout the day or as is needed.

ACCUMULATING POWER AND PROTECTION

Once you have cleansed yourself you can develop power and protection in the following manner.

The procedure is as follows:

1. Imagine yourself sitting in a circle with yourself at the centre of the circle. You also may wish to actually draw a physical circle around you as you visualize this process.
2. Now imagine that there are numerous duplicates of yourself surrounding you at the perimeter of the circle. These duplicates of yourself are beautiful, powerful and filled with energy and protection. Take time to build these images of yourself. Once you feel happy with the images of yourself looking youthful, spiritually strong and positive, filled with healing

power, see these expressions of yourself moving one by one towards you.

3. As each one merges with your body, feel yourself filling with their power, protection and healing energies. You are becoming their power and filling more and more with their light and healing.
4. Continue this until all the emanations of yourself have filled your body, and you are filled with positive energy, spiritual power and protection.

You may wish to vary this by imagining various Buddhas around you, a Spiritual friend or teacher, Reiki symbols or some other symbol which holds spiritual meaning for you.

THE MOON AND YOU, MENSTRATION AND SEXUAL ENERGY

For female of Reiki practitioners, it is important to be aware of how our bodies natural cycles effect our energy. To this end it is worth considering how one is feeling (energetically speaking), during menses. Although not formally stated in the Reiki teachings, many healing traditions of old have taken this view into account.

It is always a personal choice for a woman to use this time to go within, to give oneself, self healing and to nurture and be aware of ones energy. For this reason, some female Reiki practitioners choose to refrain from giving Reiki to others during this time.

The reasons for this lie in the knowledge that at this time a woman on her moon is purifying toxins, contaminants and lower vibrational energy from her body and energy field. This in no way is seen as a negative view, it is however important to know how this process may subtly effect healing work and the interaction of this with the human energy field. During this time the body is cleansing and purifying itself from the inner to the outer and subsequently this can in some circumstances, translate as an interference by transferring lower vibrational energy with Reiki energy to others.

This ancient knowledge is supported by many indigenous medicine cultures throughout the world and seen by some as a fundamental spiritual law. In many ways women are very fortunate to have this built in purification, where men have to deal with their own purification in other ways. The ancient tradition of the sauna in Northern Europe and the Sacred Sweatlodge Ceremony of the Native American Indian Traditions is another excellent purification process which caters for both sexes.

Further extensions to this view of menstruation held by many native traditions, is avoiding sexual intercourse for similar reasons of transference. Ultimately, the rule of thumb, is to be aware during this time and to honour, if the need arises, to go within and refrain from sexual activity during this sacred time. Another consideration for the Reiki practitioner is ones use of sexual energy. As one becomes more attuned to subtle energy, it is considered most important where one directs their sexual energy. For this reason, who one chooses to have sexual relations with is worthy of attention. If you currently are or become intimately involved with another, consider this persons energetic state. Whether one has one or numerous partners, a certain amount of energy transference occurs during sexual congress. The view is to be aware of your energy, how this affects your body and mind and to be mindful of giving your partner pleasure is respectful and loving way.

Chapter 11

'One who thinks and acts to achieve his own ends is a worldly being. One who thinks and works for others' welfare alone is a Dharma practitioner.'

— **Jamgon Kongtrul Lodro Thaye**, *Mind Training in Seven Points*

THE FIVE ELEMENTS FOR HEALING

Essentially, there are five elements to consider when facilitating Reiki for another, and they are as follows:

1. Centering
   - (a) Accessing
   - (b) Clearing
   - (c) Personal Boundaries
2. Purpose
3. Accessing
4. Treatment
5. Boundaries

CHECK LIST FOR HANDS-ON HEALING

Having explored a number of preliminary procedures,

here is the condensed procedure of beginning a session as taught in Reiki II workshop.

1. Gather information from the recipient regarding their needs.

   Ask: 'Have you had a Reiki Session before?'. If not, briefly explain the process.

   Ask: 'Is there anywhere that you require healing?'.

   Once you have a general idea of what they require, ask them to close their eyes and relax.

2. *Centering procedure*: Place your hands on your heart and close your eyes.

   Accessing: Ask inwardly with the Sei He Ki : 'Am I energetically clear?' If 'Yes' go to step 4.

3. *Clearing*: If 'No', the procedure goes as follows:

   Visualize the Sei He Ki in front of you. Now imagine this symbol in the colour blue passing through your body and energy field, purifying any areas of imbalance. Affirm in your mind as this is occurring: 'I now clear any lesser and lower energy from my body and mind, and only the highest energies remain. All is transformed into the healing power of Reiki.'

   Access again 'Am I now clear?' If yes go to step 4. If not, repeat until clear.

4. *Personal Boundaries:* Now seal your Thymus chakra with a Blue Sei He Ki, stating the name of the symbol three times. This establishes your personal boundaries throughout the healing procedure.

5. *Purpose:* State in your mind that you will remain grounded and centred throughout the procedure,

using the Hon Sha Ze Sho Nen for centering. Also, state your wish for the person receiving the healing, that they will benefit and receive all healing necessary for their highest good.

6. *Accessing:* Now place your hand on the recipient and access with the Sei He Ki. Ask inwardly:

   'Are you willing to receive this healing?' If 'Yes', continue.

   If 'No', access again asking for a direct link to the Transpersonal self. If you receive a further 'No' respect this and do not proceed. An inward 'No' does not often occur. Usually if the person has requested a session, then inwardly we receive a 'Yes'. However in the case that we do receive a definite 'No', respect this and do not proceed with the session. It simply may not be appropriate at that time.

7. *Treatment:* In your own way commence the session.

   Employ scanning techniques and internal dialogue (use Sei He Ki)

   Ask inwardly:
   - 'Where would you like my hands?'
   - 'Do you require any symbols?'
   - 'Have you had enough energy?'
   - 'Where would you like my hands next?'

8. *Personal Boundaries:* Once you feel the healing is complete, wash your hands and seal your Thymus chakra with the Sei He Ki. This disconnects you from the recipient's energy field. One can also cleanse the hands by blowing a Sei Hi Ki into the hands at the end of a session, then sealing personal boundaries.

9. Gently bring the person round and share your experiences.

   Be sure not to over interpret or diagnose their condition, we simply share what we sensed in the session.

WORKING HANDS-ON WITH REIKI II

There are a number of ways to apply Reiki on the body while facilitating healing for oneself or another. Essentially there are two approaches. The first being a sequential step by step approach and the other being intuitive. Intuitive healing comprises eight major avenues. We will explore these models here, but first a brief outline of the traditional hands on sequence from level one.

1. Traditional Hand Positions

In following the sequence of the hand positions from level I Reiki, we can visualize or draw the Cho Ku Rei where our hands are present to magnify the healing energy flowing through to the participant. This same procedure is followed for each new hand position.

2. Intuitive Healing

Here, we depart from a step by step approach and utilize a variety of approaches to access the healing methods required.

As the term suggests, we are working intuitively on where we are guided in a healing session.

In looking at most indigenous healing practitioners from around the globe, the following methods are often employed in traditional healing work. These methods use various modes of perception to obtain information regarding what is required to heal the individual, and include both psychic and clairvoyant approaches. The methods employ scanning, seeing, beaming, clearing and extracting, transmuting, infusing, smoothing, raking, and internal dialogue.

So let's map these one by one.

A. Scanning

This technique falls under the kinaesthetic mode of perception.

Here we use our hands to scan the energy field just above the body, (generally 7 cm from the body). This is usually conducted at the beginning of a session, and is facilitated from the top of the body to the bottom. The practitioner may repeat this process a number of times throughout the session or parts of it, depending upon the individual case.

As we scan, what are we looking for? The sensations that can be experienced are varied and may include a feeling of warmth or tingling in the palms, a heaviness or buldge or a strong feeling that the hands want to be placed in an area. All these sensations generally indicate a place of some description, which requires healing.

B. Seeing

This technique uses the eyes, and falls under the category of a visual mode of perception.

Here, we look down the body in a similar way to scanning. In this approach we are looking into the body and energy field. Not everyone sees auras, and in most cases we sense rather than see areas that require healing. As we look down and through the body, we may sense dull or vibrant areas in the energy field and the body. Generally dull colours indicate congestion, depletion and imbalance, whereas the vibrant colours indicate health and vitality. As part of this procedure, we imagine that we are viewing the internal organs of the body. It is almost like we are viewing each organ as if they were translucent. In using this technique, we are looking or sensing for the dull or heavy areas. You may not see these with your physical eyes as such, but rather are sensing these places. Once we have identified the depleted or diseased areas, we can begin the process of clearing these with symbols, creative visualization and Reiki energy.

C. Beaming

In this method we project healing energy from our palms to the recipient. Here the hands are held off the body. We may even be some distance from the person and with our intent, we direct this healing energy and symbols to the person and afflicted areas. This same approach can also be utilized using the eyes, directing healing energy and symbols from our eyes to the affected area, and directing healing energy from our heart chakra to the person requiring healing. Directing healing energy from the heart is particularly useful with issues to do with the giving and receiving of love, intimacy issues and for creating a feeling of safety and nurturing.

D. Clearing and Extracting

In this procedure the practitioner is removing harmful discursive energies from the individual. These can be extracted using the Cho Ku Rei in a reverse fashion, spiralling outwards, anticlockwise, and pulling the negative energy with it. This can then be transmuted, as described in the next technique. A practitioner may also remove these obstacles with both hands, as if pulling out a physical object, this can also be visualized whilst the hands are within the energy field. Another method of extracting and clearing energy is sucking the diseased energy via the mouth. This is a practice common amongst many indigenous Shamanic healers; however, this procedure is also very dangerous. With this method, the practitioner is highly susceptible to taking on this lower vibration energy, and can be greatly affected if they do not have the skill to deal with it once it is inside their body. Even amongst highly skilled native healers, the result of such methods often has a debilitating effect on the shaman, who for days or in some cases even weeks, feels the repercussions of such methods. As a general rule of thumb, don't try this particular method, as the risks are simply too high. Other methods of extracting can be used with a quartz crystal, where the lower energy is drawn into the crystal, to later be cleansed and transmuted.

A healer may also visualize the lower energy leaving the body via the lower orifices, hands or soles of the feet as black smoke, creepy crawlies or black sludge. These should be seen as leaving the body and going deep into the earth, or transmuted into positive symbols or healing energy.

E. Transmuting

In this approach, once negative energy has been extracted from the energy field, the practitioner can transmute this energy into a positive energy or simply release it. This is done using the Sei He Ki. Once the energy is drawn out using the Cho Ku Rei, it is kept in the hand and the practitioner blows or infuses a Sei He Ki, which transmutes this into positive energy. Practitioners also may visualize the harmful energy transmuting into light, diamonds, stars and the like and then proceed to place these back into the body, via the method of infusing. Lower vibration energy can also be transmuted using a bucket of salty water. Once the negative energy is removed from the body and energy field, it is thrown or projected into the salt water. The water absorbs the negative energy where the salt breaks down the negative energies and makes it neutral. Ideally using symbols and transmuting directly is the preferred method. In some healing circles, you will occasionally see a healer throw negative energy behind them on the floor, or shaking their hands as if trying to flick off something. This is another inappropriate practice, as it is a form of psychic littering. If lower vibration energy is thrown away, without the conscious intent to transmute it, it will simply hang around and transfer onto some other unsuspecting person, or even the person it was extracted from in the first place when they hop off the table after the session. This is why it is very important to transmute energy, and the more the better if it is turned into something positive.

F. Infusing

Infusing uses the breath to implant symbols into the

body, to clear meridians, chakras or through the central energy channel which runs through the centre of the body. This is propelled with a short sharp breath from the belly or Hari. The intent is to infuse a symbol into the area that requires healing. The practitioner may also use this same method for transmuting negative energy that has been extracted, and change it into a positive energy, by infusing the Sei He Ki.

G. Smoothing and Raking the Aura

Smoothing the Aura at the end of a session is a way to balance the field from the activity that has taken place during the healing. This is done with both hands, fingers together from the crown chakra to the feet, usually three consecutive times. The hands should be 7 cm from the body.

Raking the aura is a way to energize and ground the recipient after a healing. This is the same procedure as smoothing, but instead the practitioner starts at the feet and makes their way to the crown and the hands have the fingers spread wide open, much like a rake. Usually, raking is followed by smoothing at the end of a healing session. These same methods can also be applied when the person is seated after the session on the back of the person from the back of the head to the coccyx at the base of the spine and repeating this in reverse to the crown with the raking technique.

H. Internal dialogue

This technique enables a conversation using simple 'Yes/No' responses and the naming of body areas to direct healing energy. We begin by asking the question:

'What does this person require to be healed?' accessing with the Sei He Ki as mentioned in the checklist for hands-on healing.

The following is a hypothetical internal dialogue one might encounter in a healing session.

F = Facilitator of the healing

RTPS = Recipient's Transpersonal Self

For example:

F: 'Where would you like my hands?' RTPS: 'Upper chest and forehead.'

F: 'Do you require any symbols here?' RTPS: 'Cho Ku Rei and Sei He Ki.'

F: 'Have you had enough energy here?' RTPS: 'Yes.'

F: 'Where else would you like my hands next?' RTPS: 'Shoulders, etc...'

As we become more adept at these processes, we usually find that there may be a number of these modes of perception interchanging and working simultaneously. It should be pointed out that one does not simply have this ability from the outset, and it often requires practice and time to develop these abilities. Be patient and centred when trying these approaches, they will develop with time as you grow with the Reiki system.

Chapter 12

'There is no past, and there is no present, and there is no future, for even time itself is an illusion and by a single clap of the hand, it too can be returned to the void, the one experience, the timeless reality which is the mind of the Buddha.'

— ***Mikao Usui***

ABSENT HEALING ACROSS TIME AND SPACE

Absent healing is what makes Reiki II a unique level. Here we move beyond working on a physical level in this time and space, and boldly venture to new and exciting dimensions.

With Absent healing we have the ability to send healing to present situations, events and people as well as ourselves. We can also direct healing energy to past situations to affect our current outlook, and into the future to set up favourable circumstances for our lives.

In other words, we are working on a quantum level with the energy. With the dawn of quantum physics, science is just beginning to prove what mystic traditions have known since time immemorial.

So, how does it work? Using the Reiki symbols as a gateway for universal energy, we use the spiritual law of correspondence to direct energy to whichever time and space we desire.

The symbol that is the primary tool for this, is the Hon Sha Ze Sho Nen. In a way, one could look at it as a time vehicle. What this means is, that one can send healing to someone on the other side of the world and they will experience the result, as if you were physically present with them. There are no time delays, it happens in that moment, regardless of time zones in different countries.

THE QUANTUM UNIVERSE

The Webster's Dictionary describes quantum theory as: 'a theory in physics based on the concept of subdivision of radiant energy into finite quanta and applied to numerous processes involving transference or transformation of energy in an atomic or molecular scale.'

In layman's terms, this means we are all interconnected.

We live in a quantum universe, what this means is that on the subatomic level, these tiny particles (which make up the very fabric of the universe) are interconnected and unified and this unified field has intelligence. For example, a sub atomic particle will know what another subatomic particle knows on the other side of the world, or the other side of the galaxy for that matter.

This startling discovery, however, goes beyond this information with the fact that this occurs instantaneously. There are no time delays involved, and it is not a question of faster than the speed of light because it occurs instantly on a simultaneous level.

What Quantum theory suggests is that there is interconnectedness between all life and that anywhere on the scale between the macrocosm and microcosm, intelligence is present.

In the spiritual order of things this is, of course, old knowledge. It is comforting to know that science is finally understanding that consciousness is not something merely happening just in one's head, but rather is fluid and free flowing beyond the existence of time, dimension and space.

So how does this apply to absent healing? In absent healing, using symbols as a pathway on which energy can travel, we actively shape this intelligent energy from one place, time or space to another. This occurs at the same time, creating the desired result, which is the transference of healing energy.

Quantum mechanics may explain the reason why this occurs; however, what is really important here is the fact that this phenomenon does occur and it is happening all the time.

A classic example to illustrate this point is thinking of a friend and moments later they call you and say, 'I was just thinking about you', or the very next day you unexpectedly bump into them in the street.

So what's going on here? Is it merely coincidence? The answer to this is of course 'No'.

There are no mistakes in the universe, everything

happens for a reason and everything is connected to everything and this 'everything' is Universal Energy.

All we are doing with absent healing is shaping this universal energy to effect the healing outcome of another. As the understanding of this grows, so does our ability to shape this to create situations that would benefit ourselves and the lives of others.

A great percentage of people simply go through life hoping all will go smoothly and put happiness down to good luck, good karma or a favourable God smiling upon them. The difference one can make with these tools, puts the practitioner into the driver's seat of their own lives. We begin to shape our reality and to determine the outcome of events that will benefit all, by shaping Universal Intelligence using the power of our own minds. This shaping is a union between our own mind, the mind of the person involved and the Universal Energy, higher intelligence or if you like *Star Wars,* 'The Force'.

The analogy of 'The Force' as portrayed in the *Star Wars* trilogy, is a beautiful example to demonstrate Universal Energy. It suggests that the Universe is power, and that this power can have many faces. There is the good side of the Force, and the dark side of the Force, it is still the Force. What determines the kind that it is comes down to one's intent and motivation.

To work with the dark side, one simply operates out of ignorance and is driven by emotions like greed, manipulation, power over others, self-delusion, egotism and the desire to harm. To work out of the good side is to operate out of love, compassion, unity, peace, joy, healing and happiness. Essentially there is a fine line between healing and sorcery. Our vehicle is our motivation, or intentions, whether they are life giving or life destroying.

THE LAW OF CORRESPONDENCE

The Law of Correspondence works on the premise that if we use an object, effigy or proxy as a model for the healing we wish to transfer, then this will create a link to the other. This spiritual law is the basis for almost all non-local healing work. In using the Reiki symbols to form a bridge, we can effectively make a pathway for the Reiki energy to travel. This process transcends ordinary time, as it is not fixed in three dimensional time and space. The Reiki symbols go beyond the physical levels and as a result are not bound by the laws of linear time.

ABSENT HEALING PROCEDURE

The following is the procedure given to Reiki II students.

Where possible gain conscious permission from the recipient.

You will need the name and location of the person, a proxy (i.e., a teddy bear) and/or a photograph of the person.

1. Centre yourself and establish boundaries as in the checklist for hands on healing.
2. Establish permission:

   Hold both hands out in front of you and declare: 'Sei

He Ki, Sei He Ki, Sei He Ki. Name, Name, Name (person concerned) Are you there?' At this point you will get a sense of the thought form of the individual, between your hands.

State: 'Are you free to accept this healing at an appropriate time?'

If you receive a firm 'Yes', proceed.

If you receive a firm 'No', blow through your hands three times and dismiss.

Once you have a 'Yes' to the healing, STATE : At which time the healing will transfer, or if unknown: 'From the time that you go to sleep, to the time you wake up'.

3. With hands still cupped, with one hand, draw over the other:

   HON SHA ZE SHO NEN

   SEI HE KI

   CHO KU REI

4. Now transfer your cupped hands gently to the proxy.

   You are now sending healing energy, (or at the time stated), to the recipient.

5. While you are sending the energy, be open to receiving information concerning their healing.

   Ask: 'Is there anywhere you would like my hands?'

   'Do you require any symbols?', etc.

6. Send for as long as is needed, implement scanning and clearing procedures, if required.

7. Once the healing is complete, slowly move hands from the proxy, and once again cup hands in front of you.

   Draw:
   HON SHA ZE SHO NEN
   SEI HE KI
   CHO KU REI (This seals the healing.)

8. Bless and dismiss. State: 'You are now dismissed, may you be well and happy.'

   Blow through cupped hands three times.

9. Seal your Thymus chakra.

METHODS FOR ABSENT HEALING

If we look at the various ways to send an absent healing, there are essentially four methods. The following techniques can be implemented after the individual has been called in with the three symbols and the bridge drawn to the recipient.

Method 1. Using your body as a proxy

Here we use the law of correspondence, utilizing both our knees and thighs as our proxy.

In this approach we identify our right knee to correspond to the head of the recipient. Then working our way down our thigh, stating: "My upper thigh now corresponds to the recipient's upper chest", with the opposite knee and thigh corresponding to the back of the head and the upper thigh corresponding to the recipient's shoulders and upper back.

A further extension of this is to give yourself a treatment, with the hand positions and your body corresponding to the person you are sending to. In this way we are facilitating a Reiki self-treatment, as well as sending absent healing to another.

Method 2. Using a teddy bear as a proxy

With this method, instead of using your body as a proxy, we use a teddy bear to represent the individual receiving the healing. This method is a good extension when facilitating absent healing on the inner child or issues from the past.

Another extension is to use a pillow or pillows on a massage table, much like a mannequin, and to commence a full treatment as if the person was lying on the massage table.

Anything can be used as a proxy, i.e., a handbag, a rolled up sweater, a crystal, etc. Using the law of correspondence, we can apply this method to anything as a proxy.

Method 3. Cupped hands

Here we use the space between our cupped hands and visualize that our hands are now holding a certain area of the body. This technique works particularly well for healing issues or for manifesting goals. In addition to this, we can also use this method as a way to work on the inner organs of the body. For example: "My hands are now holding the heart of the recipient."

Method 4. Visualization

In this method we simply visualize ourselves healing the individual. We visualize that we are present with them and that they are receiving hands on healing from ourselves. This technique requires greater mental focus, so it is suggested not to have any outside distractions where possible.

SENDING HEALING ENERGY TO A SITUATION

Sending Reiki to a situation that requires resolve or healing is another way to work with absent healing. The process is the same procedure as before, the only difference being the 'calling in' stage. In this stage we state the situation clearly and precisely three times until we feel contact with the issue between our hands. Then we follow the usual procedure as in the checklist for absent healing. For example: I am now calling: 'The healing resolve between myself and Amanda, The healing resolve between myself and Amanda', etc., stating the intent three times.

SENDING HEALING TO MORE THAN ONE PERSON

Group healing is a way to be more effective in your healing because you can effectively be in more than one place at once.

What this requires, is an individual 'calling in' procedure, and the signing of the three symbols which creates a bridge to not only one individual, but to many.

The procedure is as follows:

After establishing boundaries and setting your intent for healing, call in each person by name and location, and sign the three symbols on each person. This can be in the form of an individual photograph or individual piece of paper with the person's details on it. Once you have called in all the individuals concerned, move your hands to a proxy of your choice, stating that this proxy corresponds to all the individuals in the photographs. Send for approximately 10 to 20 minutes and close with one bridge to ignite the process: Hon Sha Ze Sho Nen, Sei He Ki, Cho Ku Rei, and blow through cupped hands.

Effectively, each individual called in has received the required amount of energy. In directing the healing, it is best to do the full traditional hand positions, as that way you'll cover all areas required in the treatment of so many.

A common misconception that one may assume from this procedure, is the question, "If the energy is infinite, why can't I just send a healing to one hundred people and sign the bridge once?"

This approach will work; however in this case, the recipients will only receive 1% of the universal energy sent. It is essential to call in each three symbols for each individual to be 100% effective in the transmission of the healing. This same law also applies for initiation procedures.

THE REIKI BOX

Another excellent way to send absent healing to many individuals, or wide scale situations like natural disasters, accidents, countries in conflict, political unrest, etc., is to send healing using the Reiki Box.

In this procedure, the practitioner needs a small box preferably made of natural materials. Contained within the box is the people or situations that require healing.

In order to be most effective, each situation or person must be called in by signing the three Reiki II symbols over each person. Photos of the individuals are useful; however, if they are not available then the recipients' full names and where they live will suffice. Once all are called in, we send healing to the box, with each hand either side sending healing energy to the situations and people needing healing.

A more general approach is to call everyone into the box at the calling in stage, not stating all the names, just a general invocation. Here we draw the symbols once for all the beings concerned. This simplified version sends just one stream of energy to the group instead of many, so for example if there were 10 people's names or photos in the box, then each person would only receive 10% each of the healing energy. This method works particularly well for geographical locations which require healing, like the Amazon forest or a country at war.

As the box is used on a continual basis, the energy will build more and more. These boxes can really be a beacon of healing energy in themselves. After some time, a person need only put a photo in the box for that individual to receive healing energy and a blessing. It is for this reason that natural materials are recommended, as they hold and accumulate energy better than synthetic materials.

SENDING HEALING TO OUR INNER CHILD

Most of our adult lives are lived out of our conditioned experience from childhood. This occurs usually in our formative years, approximately from birth until age 7. It is at this age that we form base concepts of our outer world, in particular, how to receive affection and love and the ways to achieve this basic human need. It is often from the denial of love that stems our wounding and resultantly, our dysfunctional responses that we live out in our relationships and interactions with people as adults.

Sending healing to the archetype of our inner child can be rewarding, sometimes confronting and often insightful in the healing of old patterns.

The procedure follows the same practice as before, with the only variation being the calling in stage. For example: After accessing with the Sei He Ki, calling : "Myself at age five, myself at age five, myself at age five, Am I there?" Then proceeding with the three symbols to bridge the healing.

It is generally suggested that people use a teddy bear as a proxy, as this symbolically represents holding yourself as the child. This process can often bring up varied emotional responses in people; such as: tears, sadness, joy or play. Most people report that this practice is a very gentle way to touch a deep part of our innocence. It is very healing to hold ourselves as children, and comfort the unloved parts of ourselves.

A further extension of this is to send an absent healing to your inner child, with each day representing a year of your life, and to repeat this each day consecutively till your current age. In effect you are healing your life. In doing this for each consecutive year, the energy squares itself and becomes an accumulation of power each day.

The only drawback is, the older you are in years, the longer this process will take to complete.

SENDING HEALING TO PAST ISSUES

Sending healing to the past is a beneficial way to heal current issues that we hold in our lives now, or for the healing of another's issues. Within the first seven years of our lives we form many of the foundations of our conditioning for this lifetime.

The method used here is the calling in of an issue and stating that the healing energy be sent to the origin of the issue. During the procedure, the practitioner will state: 'I am now sending healing energy to the root cause of the issue I have with (state the issue).' This is stated three times and healing energy is sent to this time. Now with this procedure, we do not need to know the year the issue was formed, because by simply calling in the origin of the issue and bridging with the symbols, the Divine Intelligence of the Reiki energy will go to that time and heal whatever is most appropriate.

In other cases, we may know the specific date, month or year that an agenda was formed, and if this is the case, we call in this time as our reference point.

A question that sometimes comes up with regard to healing past issues, 'Why can't I send healing to all my issues from the past that affect me now, in one healing?' The response to this is, yes you can, but the effectiveness of your approach would be like trying to melt an iceburg with a magnifying glass. The more appropriate approach is to send healing to specific issues, and perhaps work on an issue every day for several days. Sometimes one healing is sufficient to heal an issue, and other times it is an ongoing process. By specializing in a particular area, we pull all our resources into one place and our effectiveness is, therefore, much greater.

SENDING HEALING ENERGY INTO THE FUTURE

When sending healing into the future, we apply the same principles and methods used to send healing to the past. The only difference is the calling stage and what is stated. If, for example, we were wanting to send absent healing to a court case for ourselves or someone else, we could do the following: We could send healing to the judge so that he would be in a good and moral space, and to each person at the hearing. If we didn't know exactly what time of the day the hearing was, then all that is required, is to state that the energy activates the moment you walk into the court room or words to this effect. It is sufficient to direct healing energy into the future and it is not necessary to know the specific linear time or location for that matter. It can, therefore, be activated by a cue of some kind.

Another example would be sending healing energy to a future exam, so that you would be calm, clear and recall all the material necessary. If perhaps the exam is delayed or postponed for another day, then the energy simply carries over to when a specific cue is put in place. Your cue for example, could be when you pick up your pen at the beginning of the exam, and then the energy is activated for your highest good.

Sending healing to the future can bring together all the elements in a situation to work in your favour. This is by no means the manipulation of circumstances, as the Reiki energy is always set with the highest intent: 'For the benefit of all concerned', or, 'This or something better be done'.

Through sending healing energy and symbols to future events, we remove any obstacles that prevent flow, thus, promoting creative evolution and harmony.

Some other examples of future situations are: to send healing to a journey, flight or car ride, a business meeting, a seminar, a job interview, a holiday, a party, a wedding, a funeral, a work environment, etc.

Sending healing to future events also secures a location from any negative influences that may otherwise create a disturbance in the natural order of things.

SENDING HEALING TO SITUATIONS OF CONFLICT AND CRISES

Absent healing can be invaluable in times of great distress, anxiety or emergencies. Often-times when we are faced with dire circumstances, we don't know what to do.

In these situations we can apply absent healing, even if we are not present or even know the individual(s) involved. An example of this may be driving past a road accident. We simply call in the situation, all the people concerned, even if we don't know the name, it is enough to state: "The woman injured in the crash", stating this three times and using the symbols to bridge the healing. Another example may be when we see a person in distress or feeling anxiety. In doing so we are sending pure unconditional love to soothe and calm the person concerned.

A Personal Experience:

I was travelling on a train one day and an elderly woman boarded the train just before it took off. The woman hadn't had time to find a seat when the train took off suddenly, the woman fell hard on the floor and broke her hip. A young man nearby came immediately to her aid. I was at the other end of the train but could see what had happened. Rather than crowd the poor lady as others were doing, I immediately sent absent healing to her via the coat that was sitting on my knees as the proxy. As soon as my hands touched the coat, tremendous heat filled my hands and the healing began to transfer. As an ambulance was being called, I could see that the man who had originally came to her aid had his hands on her the whole time. Seeing as he was comforting her during the whole ordeal, I gave him a temporary Reiki I alignment as a visualization with the same proxy, channelling this healing energy in two streams. Once the alignment was complete he was then performing Reiki for the woman. She seemed much calmer as a result and kept looking at me as though she knew that I was helping her in some way.

After the ambulance had taken her away, I had the opportunity to speak to the man who had come to her aid. He spoke about his experience and he felt that there was a higher force working through him, and that he had felt a heat in his hands. After explaining to him what this force was, he was very thankful and excited, and wished to know more about how to further this ability. The thing to note here is that without his knowledge, the Reiki energy was activated in him as a temporary alignment, and healing energy was facilitated to benefit another.

This is further explained in chapter 18 on Absent attunements.

SENDING ABSENT HEALING TO TWO PEOPLE AT THE SAME TIME

This procedure uses the body as a proxy to direct healing energy to two people simultaneously. The practice is ideal for relationships in conflict, whether they be between couples, a father and son, a falling out between friends, etc.

The Procedure:

1. Follow the usual procedures of setting up boundaries and centring.

2. Using both hands, calling in the first individual, stating their name three times and once you have a connection, sign or visualize the three symbols in sequence.
3. Using your body as the proxy, now transfer this energy to your left knee.
4. Remembering that one part of your body needs to maintain contact throughout the absent healing procedure, slide your elbow down to your knee to maintain your contact and to free up your hands for the next stage.
5. Now with your hands free once again, yet still leaning your elbow on your left knee (which is person one). Call in the second person in the traditional manner, three times, establish connection and sign or visualize the three symbols.
6. Now transfer the second person to your right knee as the proxy.
7. Slide your left hand down to your knee once again.
8. Now think to your self that one knee represents one individual, and your other knee represents the other person. As long as one hand is on the proxy, healing energy is being sent simultaneously or two streams of energy.
9. Turn your attention to your left knee and using internal dialogue ask the question, 'what does this person need to heal the conflict at hand?' (state the situation).

   Sign whichever symbols come and direct healing energy to the person, imagining the areas where they are carrying the emotional pain of the conflict.

10. Repeat this process for the other person in a similar manner.
11. Once both people have received all they require, gently lift both hands off your knees together and place your hands cupped together at your heart centre. Here we are combining the two individuals together and reuniting them.
12. Now sign the Sei He Ki three times with both hands or simply visualize this between your hands and infuse this with a Cho Ku Rei. (The Sei He Ki activates the highest healing outcome.)
13. Sign any additional symbols you feel appropriate. Once you feel the healing is complete, sign the three symbols in the standard closing procedure and blow through your cupped hands three times to release the healing.

This procedure directly removes the root cause of conflict between two people, if you like, it removes the fuel from the fire. Without the cause of the conflict present, this bridges differences and makes the way to a peaceful and harmonious resolution. This procedure may also be repeated a number of times in serious issues of conflict.

COMBINING ABSENT HEALING WITH HANDS ON PROCEDURES

In this practice, we can effectively work on issues surrounding a present situation from the past.

A person may come to you requiring healing on an

injury from the past that causes regular pain. So an example could be to work on the affected area and while you are sending healing to this physical part, call in the original injury three times, and sign or visualize the three symbols as a bridge to the injury's origin. Once this contact is made, use this point on the body as your proxy. This way healing energy is being sent to the current issue, as well as another time and space, in this case healing the actual injury itself. This assists in the releasing of the trauma that the body experienced, as well as the psychological and emotional pain and stress endured at that time, effectively being in two places at once.

We can also apply this same procedure for emotional pain or childhood abuse issues, fears and phobias, etc. The beauty of these techniques is that the recipient does not need to re-experience the pain and trauma all over again; the energy simply goes to these places and gently heals these issues.

~ Chapter 13 ~

'It is the wish of Wakan Tanka, (The Creator), that the light enters the darkness that we may see not only with our two eyes, but the one eye which is of the heart and with which we see and know all that is true and good.'

— ***Black Elk***

REIKI AND CRYSTALS

As mentioned previously Crystals are dualistic in nature. So before using a crystal in healing, there are a number of important factors to recognise. These are as follows:

- The type of crystal
- The purification of the crystal
- The programming of the crystal
- How to use crystals for Absent Healing
- The maintenance and energetic care of the crystal.

It is vitally important to consider these points before we use a crystal to be sure that all the safeguards are in place, to bring about the highest intent for healing.

The Type of Crystal

Quartz based crystals are generally best for healing work, especially clear quartz.

The size of the crystal is not that important, it is more the case to find a crystal that you connect with and feels right for you.

Purification of the Crystal

Once you have a crystal you are happy with, you will need to cleanse it from previous people who have handled it or programmed it. A crystal is like a sponge and absorbs energy from its surrounding environment.

To purify a crystal, use natural spring water or better still a natural spring, river or lake. One can use water and natural earth to wash the crystal or place it in the earth. A common misconception is using salt water to cleanse a crystal. Quartz Crystals don't grow out of the ocean, so it makes sense to use elements that are natural to a crystal's environment. Salt water can be quite damaging to the energy field of the crystal and should be avoided when possible.

Once we have purified the crystal in water, we can energize the crystal on a full moon overnight. This will energize the crystal and establish a balance with the energies of sky and earth.

The Programming of the Crystal for Absent Healing

Hold the crystal in your hands and clear the crystal once again, using the clearing exercise from the check-list for hands on healing. Passing the Sei He Ki through the crystal three times, stating that any lesser or lower energies now leave this crystal and only the highest energies remain, all is transformed into the highest good.

Now we are ready to programme the crystal with any intent we desire.

Sign the three symbols as in an absent healing: Hon Sha Ze Sho Nen, Sei He Ki, Cho Ku Rei. Now state clearly and precisely your intent for the crystal, stating this three times and blowing a Cho Ku Rei into the crystal after each intent stated.

Once you feel this is complete, sign the three symbols again and blow through the crystal and cupped hands three times. This activates the programme.

How to Use Crystals for Absent Healing

Using crystals is especially good for absent healing, as they magnify the Reiki energy. If you have a crystal for absent healing, use it as the proxy and keep the purpose of the crystal only for healing work. This will build up the intent over time and contain the energy for that specific purpose.

Using crystals on the body or in hands on sessions is generally an unnecessary extension to traditional Reiki. It is important not to rely on external tools and props. All that we need to facilitate Reiki is supplied on our body: two hands, a mind and an open heart.

Keep the use of crystals and Reiki covert if you intend to use them.

Someone who has not been exposed to Reiki before could get the wrong impression that, "Reiki, oh yeah that's all about using crystals for healing."

Also avoid using crystal layouts on the body in your healing work, it is vitally important to have a solid knowledge on how the crystal's energy field interacts with the human energy field.

Unless you have a complete knowledge of this practice, it is best to leave it alone.

Ideally, we should be presenting Reiki in a way that holds true to the original practice. If you are intent on using crystals as an exploration, you can keep one in your pocket or near you, as this will amplify your energy field while you are practicing Reiki.

Care and Maintenance of an Absent Healing Crystal

It is best to only let yourself handle the crystal, to keep the vibrations aligned to your energy field. This is not for any superstitious reason, it is merely a way to keep the energies of the crystal aligned with your field.

A way to maintain your crystal is to cleanse it after your absent healings with either a Smudge Stick (Sage smoke), or by using the Sei He Ki clearing exercise. In addition to this, it is good to leave your crystal under moonlight in nature every month, to allow it to absorb the frequencies from the elements of nature.

Chapter 14

'Without leaving the house, one may know all there is in heaven and earth. Without peeping from the window, one may see the ways of heaven. Those who go out learn less and less the more they travel. Wherefore does the sage know all without going anywhere, see all without looking, do nothing and yet achieve.'

— ***Lao Tzu***, *Tao Te Ching*

THE CHAKRAS

The word Chakra (Sanskrit), Cakkhu (Pali) means: wheel, centre, eye, energy nexus within the subtle energy body. The chakras are the basis of the energetic structure of the human being. These energy centres stem along a central axis point (central channel) that runs from the crown chakra to three finger widths below the navel.

The chakras are a vital link to the totality of our being. Each centre represents a mirrored aspect of who we are. Working with these sources of power can assist in our personal growth, well-being and personal development.

Each chakra vibrates at a specific frequency and are affected by light, colour and sound. The chakras can be affected by these means and other vibrational frequencies. These frequencies affect the chakras by means of sympathetic resonance.

The chakra system also corresponds to the endocrine system of the body. The endocrine system controls the hormonal balance within human beings and it is these hormones which have a strong effect on our emotions as individuals.

If our chakras are out of balance, then this will also effect our endocrine system and as a result, our emotional body. This is why chakra balancing can be very beneficial in balancing the body, mind and emotions.

There are many schools of thought about the chakras. In this example we will illustrate the system that is a common model in eastern spiritual traditions.

This system also works specifically to the Universal Reiki system.

THE CHAKRA SYSTEM

1. The Base Chakra

The base chakra is situated at the base of the body at the perineum muscle. The base chakra governs the supply of energy to the reproductive organs, the kidneys, the adrenal glands and spinal column. The base chakra relates to our will to live, survival, procreation, family law, fight-flight response and our basic human instincts. The corresponding colour is red.

2. The Sacral Chakra (Hara or Hari Chakra)

This chakra is situated three finger widths below the

belly button and protudes from the front and back of the body. It is related to our emotions of sensuality and sexuality. The sacral is related to our drive in the physical world, and supplies our immune system and sexual organs with additional power. The sacral chakra is the seat of our personal power. The corresponding colour is orange.

3. The Solar Plexus Chakra

The solar plexus chakra is situated where the rib cage meets in the lower chest. Like the sacral chakra, it protrudes from the front and back of the body. This chakra is related to issues of personal power, self-esteem/self image and our emotional selves. It is linked to the gall bladder, the digestive system and the pancreas. The corresponding colour is yellow.

4. The Heart Chakra

The heart chakra is located in the centre of our chest, this centre governs our ability to give and receive love. Here is the seat of compassion, giving, self-sacrifice, and unconditional love. The heart chakra governs the heart, the thymus gland, the circulatory system and lungs. The corresponding colour is green or pink.

4 a. The Thymus Chakra

The thymus chakra is located five finger widths above the heart chakra and just below the collarbones. This is the area of our personal boundaries and where we take in energy from our outer world. It protrudes from the thymus gland at the front of the body and emerges from C7 or the raised or protruding lump at the back of our lower neck, where our neck and shoulders meet. This centre governs our immune system and ability to ward off negative influences energetically and psychically. The associated colour is aqua or sky blue.

5. **The Throat Chakra**

The throat chakra is located in the centre of the throat and protrudes from back and front of the neck. This centre governs communication and our ability to speak our truth or to voice our opinion. The corresponding colour is deep blue.

6. **The Brow Chakra**

This chakra is located at the centre of our brow, between our eyebrows and the original hairline. This chakra protrudes from the front and back of the head and governs our intuition and intellect. It is the active centre of our imagination and our abilities of clairvoyance and psychic sensitivity. This chakra also relates to our pituitary and pineal glands. The corresponding colour is indigo.

7. **The Crown Chakra**

The crown chakra is located eight finger widths from the original hairline and is directly vertical to the tips of the ears when drawn directly upwards. The crown chakra governs our attributes of spiritual potential and universal understanding. Other related factors include, wisdom, clarity, oneness, unity and the interconnectedness with all life. It is our source to life and the activation point of the Reiki energy. The corresponding colours are purple, gold or white.

CHAKRA BALANCING

Balancing the Chakras with the Reiki symbols

The chakras or energy centres of the body are major storehouses of information relating to our physical, psychological, emotional, and psycho-spiritual selves. In relation to healing, the chakras give us a clear map of the overall health of a person on an energetic level.

During a session we may need to balance a chakra or a series of chakras.

Applying symbols and energy to each individual chakra, we greatly assist in creating balance throughout the energy body.

Procedure:

1. Draw HON SHA ZE SHO NEN over the chakra.
2. Draw SEI HE KI over the chakra.
3. Draw CHO KU REI over the chakra.

- Place palm over palm, doubling the hand chakras over each energy centre.
- Visualize each symbol (steps 1 to 3) and leave hands at the chakra point for approximately 5 minutes.
- Now repeat the whole process for each chakra centre.

It is recommended that the practitioner access the recipient with the Sei He Ki to determine whether the person has received enough energy at each point. During a session it may be that only a few points may require balancing, however as a sequence, this procedure aligns the individual and deeply touches the core of each centre and our being.

Chakra balancing may be approached from the crown to feet or from feet to crown. Be sure to access to see what is most appropriate for each individual.

This is a very powerful technique for balancing the chakras. It can be used instead of a full treatment or for one's self-healing. It can also be combined into your hands on sessions and absent healing procedures.

To finish a session, ground your client by gently massaging both feet and allow them some time to come round.

CHAKRA BALANCING AS A SELF-TREATMENT

The same procedure that we use on another can also be applied to ourselves. This process deepens our connection with our centre and establishes a deep calm throughout the process.

As we are working on the energy centres, many people report a difference in the feelings and results of these sessions. Many people report a greater depth achieved through the hands on sessions and a centredness which follows, often for days.

LIFE MAPPING THROUGH THE CHAKRAS

This method is a direct way of healing the underlying issues that shape the way we act and react in our lives.

Through the techniques of body focusing and hands on healing, we can ascertain the dominant issues in each energy centre and actively change our relationship to these issues.

This process is facilitated by breath work, body awareness and internal dialogue to pinpoint the issue in mind.

This technique is useful when we are faced with obstacles which are unknown or obscured by our emotions. It is also a good method for times when we need renewed clarity and direction in our healing path. The process is as follows:

1. This exercise involves two people, a facilitator and a recipient.
2. The recipient lies down with their eyes closed and relaxes, and the facilitator sits beside the person with a note pad and pen.
3. Now the facilitator asks the recipient to breathe into and focus their awareness on their base chakra. The recipient places their hands on their base chakra, hands on the pubic bone, palm over palm as in the chakra balancing technique. The recipient breathes into this area. The facilitator asks the recipient to ask inwardly 'Am I safe?' or 'How can I be safe?'
4. The recipient is then asked to speak whatever sense impressions come to mind in relation to the question. These can be images, thoughts, feelings, sensations, dialogue, etc. The idea is to speak the immediate impressions without analyzing them. The process encourages intuitive responses.

5. As the recipient speaks these impressions, the facilitator writes them down for future reference, making sure to clarify and read back anything which was not heard clearly.

6. A few sentences is sufficient and the facilitator directs the recipient to drop the awareness in this area and to turn their focused awareness on their sacral chakra or Hari. Following the same process as before, the recipient places their hands on their Hari. The facilitator asks the question: 'What is my personal power?' or 'Do I know and use my personal power effectively?' Speaking their immediate impressions, the facilitator writes these impressions down as before.

7. This process is repeated for the following chakras with the key questions being:

   Solar Plexus chakra: 'Am I worthy?' or 'How can I be worthy?'

8. Heart chakra: 'Do I give and receive love?' or 'How can I give and receive love?'

9. Throat chakra: 'Do I express myself?' or 'How can I express myself?'

10. Brow chakra: 'What do I need to know?' or 'Do I know what is necessary for me?'

11. Crown chakra: 'What is my spiritual path?' or 'How can I pursue my spiritual path?'

Once the facilitator has moved through this process, the recipient remains with their eyes closed and relaxed and the recipient reads back what was spoken. As this is being done, the recipient places their hands on the corresponding chakras with their hands, and adds any further impressions that may arise from these areas.

Once this is complete, the recipient looks at the information and, together the recipient and facilitator try to encapsulate these sentences into one phrase or word that summarizes the impressions. The idea is to contain each chakra with a particular phrase or 'key code'; meaning the key to unlock the code lying within the chakra. In mapping the chakras in this way, the individual has a direct insight into their overall energetic make up. Some energy centres may be negative in their summary, and some may be life-giving and positive.

When this process of elimination has determined the issue, you are left with working issues to apply hands on, absent healing or the healing triad as explained in chapter 16.

Employing the healing triad, the facilitator directs healing energy to the cause of the issue that has been disclosed through the life mapping technique. Please refer to the methods of the healing triad to complete this process.

Chapter 15

Setting up your own Reiki practice

After successfully completing traditional Reiki II, many students take the first steps towards setting up their own Reiki practice. The following suggestions are some helpful guidelines for setting up your personal practice.

- Consider how you will promote yourself, advertising, flyers, information evenings, presentations and talks, editorials in magazines, health and lifestyle expos or referral in conjunction with other health practitioners.
- Consider having an established and professional room to work from. You may consider hiring a room or working from home. Is the space you have at home conducive to a healing environment? Or would leasing a room be more appropriate for your practice?
- Will you have personal liability insurance?
- Charging an appropriate fee for your services.

As part of being a practitioner, it is wise to consider how one conducts themselves in a healing situation. At all times it is best to present yourself and your art in a professional and clear way. When we are facilitating a session for another we always endeavour to make that person as comfortable as possible. Part of this is to convey clearly what we are presenting and what they might expect from the session. A simple thing to ask once you have explained the process, is if they have any questions. This gives the recipients the opportunity to probe deeper and it will also confirm for you that they have at least a basic understanding and what role they play in their healing process.

Please refer to the AIRT Code of ethics in chapter 20. These simple codes are a solid foundation and guide to the practice of Reiki.

CREATING A SPACE CONDUCIVE TO HEALING

When circumstances permit, it is ideal to set up a room that is tailored to your Reiki practice.

Rooms that help generate positive energy are generally, well-lit with natural sun light, well-ventilated, i.e., with windows and are uncluttered in their arrangement. A simple, ordered and clean room will naturally attract positive influences. To enhance this further, you may wish to set up an altar of sacred objects that have meaning for you, often a candle and incense is a nice touch.

Setting a shrine gives a focus of intent to a room and will naturally enhance the vibration you are working with. The idea is to keep it simple. Less is more!

Before commencing a session, be sure to take the phone off the hook and let others that may be sharing your space with you know that you will need the allotted time to be relatively quiet.

If you have any pets, take them out of the room, as animals love Reiki and may distract.

To help maintain this energy between clients, smudging is also of great benefit. You can find smudge sticks at most new age shops. They are herbs wrapped in cotton that are lit and allowed to smoulder. Using the smoke from the smouldering herbs, we pass this around the room to clear any negative energy.

Be sure to open a window or door to allow the old energy to release.

The recommendations prescribed are only a guide. These methods help to support a Reiki session but they are not completely essential to be effective in your treatments. Reiki can be done anywhere and at anytime, regardless of disturbing influences in an environment, the healing taking place is still the same. Don't limit the time or places where you practice Reiki. Sometimes circumstances prevent the perfect settings being available to facilitate healing, the idea is to do the best with what you have in any given moment.

BEING CLEAR ON WHAT YOU ARE OFFERING

The point of informing clients about what you are doing is important with regard to holding true to the original

Reiki tradition. As practitioners of Reiki, part of this responsibility is not only to heal, but also to educate. This is why we need to present ourselves to the public with a view that supports the traditional system, so as not to confuse the somewhat clouded perception of Reiki.

If for example, we want to use crystals or work in the Aura, it is important to inform your client that this is not part of Reiki, but rather an extension to the healing practice. Making clear distinctions between what is Reiki and what is being incorporated into the modality, is a responsibility each Reiki practitioner holds.

HOW MUCH TO CHARGE?

Many people feel uncomfortable with charging a set rate for their healing services. It is hard to set a price on universal healing. Another way to look at this is in terms of our time and energy. To facilitate a Reiki session we need to set aside time and create a space for our prospective client, as well as preparing both mentally and psychically for the session. Most practitioners charge the same as a regular massage therapist. If however you feel uncomfortable with this, facilitating Reiki for some other service or exchange is also a nice way to go. The bottom line is to value this sacred gift, and to value ourselves as a vehicle for this energy. It is also important to recognize our concepts of abundance and the values we place on ourselves. There is no spiritual law that says we need to be a spiritual martyr. At the end of the day, time is money and we still have to pay the bills.

REIKI II CHECKLIST

1. One Reiki II Initiation, preferably at the beginning of a workshop.
2. The three Reiki II symbols are given, explained, practiced and memorized throughout the workshop.
3. At least one full hands on session using the symbols during the workshop.
4. Methods of Absent healing are explored and practiced in a variety of forms.
5. Chakras are explained and chakra balancing is practiced, one session each.
6. Using symbols to clear rooms is explained, demonstrated and practiced.
7. Personal boundaries, clearing and related centring procedures are demonstrated and practiced.
8. Practice requirements are given during and after the workshop.
9. Explanation of the Reiki II initiation and its empowerment of the Reiki II symbols.
10. Students receive a manual of procedures, symbols and techniques.
11. Students receive a certificate in second degree Reiki upon completion.
12. Total workshop duration: 12 hours.

Chapter 16

'Miracles are fantastic events which utilize hidden laws of nature that most people are not aware of. Miracles do not break the laws of nature, they are actually based on them.'

— ***Master Choa Kok Sui***

ADVANCED REIKI

Extensions and explorations beyond the traditional Reiki II level

At the Australian Institute for Reiki Training we offer an additional level between second and third degree, which although is not a traditional level, has proven to be very beneficial in fine-tuning and extending on the principles taught in Reiki levels I and II.

In Advanced Reiki we extend beyond Reiki II into areas such as:

- Clairvoyance, intuitive and psychic healing.
- Working in the human energy field (aura).
- Buddhist perspectives on death and dying.
- Buddhist archetypes for healing (Medicine Buddha, meditation and practice).
- Absent healing for numerous situations (the healing triad).

- Working with inner guidance and extending healing methods on more expansive levels.

Advanced Reiki was implemented as a workshop to explore Reiki in its myriad forms. As there is often not enough time to devote to all the areas and ways that Reiki can be applied in a seminar, this seminar offers the students the ground to explore these additional practices and methods and, in so doing, further their knowledge and practice of the healing arts. This workshop is also a useful addition for Reiki students who already combine Reiki with other modalities.

To stress once again, Advanced Reiki is not a traditional Reiki level, rather an extension and elaboration of material from the second degree Reiki system.

In the following chapter we will explore some of these methods and how these can benefit an established practitioner.

THE QUANTUM HEALING BANK

As the name suggests, this refers to stored healings and symbols that can be accessed at will or activated at specific times during healing sessions or at times when we need additional healing energy.

Because the Hon Sha Ze Sho Nen enables healing to be directed over time and space, effectively we can put a time delay on healings and their transmission in the Quantum healing bank to be activated at a time that is most appropriate for the individual receiving.

The Quantum healing bank is best imagined as a bubble or energy field above one's head, that contains an abundance of healing energy and Reiki symbols.

Some of the applications of the Quantum Healing Bank:

1. Reiki symbols can be stored for direct use by the practitioner during a healing session or in Absent healing which can be activated in the past, present or future situations.
2. Healings can be activated for oneself or another at specific times, using the Reiki Absent healing sequence.
3. Healings can be duplicated and repeated over a series of days, weeks, etc.
4. Healings or symbols can be directed to particular locations for a future time and space or for past situations.
5. The individual can consciously request healing energy at any time when they require an individual boost of positive energy, healing or protection.

How to set up a Quantum Healing Bank

1. State the person's name three times and sign the Sei He Ki.
2. Determine how many symbols or how much healing energy is required and state when this will activate.
3. Seal this intent with a Cho Ku Rei.

An Example:

Internally the dialogue is as follows: Visualize drawing the Sei He Ki. 'John, John, John, Do you require any additional healing or symbols?'

Recipient: 'Yes, healing every evening from the time that I go to sleep to the time that I wake up, for the following three nights.'

Facilitator: 'May this be for your highest good', visualize drawing a Cho Ku Rei.

To seal this intent, you may blow the Cho Ku Rei or infuse this into or just above the crown of the recipient, or visualize this being infused with the Cho Ku Rei at the end of establishing the Quantum Healing Bank.

Note: The Quantum Healing Bank needs to be attended to on a regular basis. For example, one could not set up a Quantum healing bank, for themselves to receive healings every night at a specific time for the rest of their lives. The focus for the bank is to focus healing intent, and the bank is a storage facility and vehicle for this energy transmission. Ideally for ongoing healings, the bank should be set up once or twice a week.

THE REIKI II BOOSTER ATTUNEMENT

At the Australian Institute for Reiki Training, each Reiki level has a Booster attunement, which can be facilitated by an empowered teacher to enhance a student's energy flow. This is not to say that once a student has an initiation that over time, this energy begins to dissipate, rather, the Booster attunement serves as a way of experiencing the divine power of the Reiki energy and to enhance the energy flow within the person's energy field.

During a Reiki attunement, a tremendous amount of positive healing energy is bestowed upon and through an individual, so with this in mind, receiving a Booster attunement is a direct way to enhance our field resonance.

The Reiki II Booster attunement, serves this end by activating the three Reiki symbols which are given at the Reiki II level. Receiving and giving attunements, no matter at which level, is also an empowering and pleasant experience as we are touched each time by the spiritual power and blessing of the Reiki energy.

RELEASING THE TIES THAT BIND

Releasing the ties that bind is a unique process to release oneself or another from situations of conflicts, old relationships or resentments. It is also applicable for people who have died where there are unresolved issues or never a chance to say goodbye.

This process allows forgiveness to follow as one is psychically, energetically and emotionally released from a situation.

There are often times in life where we hold on to past experiences, relationships or loved ones which have far exceeded their use by date, yet we feel bound to these feelings. Some of these factors may be purely emotional, other times, it is the energy ties which are actually still connected to our energy body, that we feel tugging at our heart strings. On occasion, it can be the experience where someone else is invading our psychic space and we need to remove this presence and re-establish our personal boundaries.

The following process assists in all of the above examples and is a direct way to release ourselves from situations that oppress us.

The procedure is as follows:

1. Call in the person as in the absent healing procedure.
2. Call the person's name three times, cupping your hands and draw or visualize: Hon Sha Ze Sho Nen, Sei He Ki, Cho Ku Rei.
3. Once you have established a connection, transfer this thought form to a proxy of your choice. (You may want to transfer this to a piece of paper.)
4. State the situation three times, detailing the issues and your desired resolve.
5. Now state the following: (state the person's name three times) 'I fully and freely release you and let you go to the Divine Intelligence, whose perfect work is in you and flows through you. I forgive you and I forgive myself. I am free and you are free and all is cleansed and released between us both, now and in the future.'
6. Sign in the air in front of you a large Sei He Ki. Imagine this is cutting the ties, visualized as cords of energy between you and the person concerned.
7. Now repeat steps 4 to 6.
8. Repeat steps 4 to 6 once more.
9. Once you have completed this sequence three times, visualize this person/situation symbolically fading off into the distance or reducing in size until

it has completely disappeared. Give thanks in your own way for the release of this situation and the lessons that were presented at the time.

10. Now burn the paper that was your proxy, stating that no harm comes to the individual concerned.
11. Close the absent healing in the traditional manner, drawing the Hon Sha Ze Sho Nen, Sei He Ki and Cho Ku Rei, blowing through cupped hands three times to complete the healing process.

This technique may be repeated on a regular basis or until the issue subsides.

HEALING TRIADS

The Healing Triad is an extension on the concepts of absent healing. It incorporates Sacred Geometry, the Cho Ku Rei, the elements of the situation, its outcome and the outer forces that come into play.

Healing Triads are particularly useful in addressing situations where there is more than one person involved, to actively remove obstacles to one's healing.

Healing Triads can be used in three ways; as an absent healing procedure; using a particular mudra (hand gesture), and visualization or a physical proxy; or applying this to the geometry of the physical body. To follow the latter example, the student can effectively facilitate absent healing on the recipient whilst performing a hands on session. But first, let's deal with the absent healing procedure.

Absent Healing Triad

The procedure is as follows:

1. Think of an issue or obstacle in your life, have a reasonable sized piece of paper and a pen.
2. Draw a large triangle on the page, big enough for you to put your hands in. Physically draw a Cho Ku Rei inside the triangle at each corner.
3. Now write these issues or what you wish to manifest, in a clear and direct manner at the centre of the triangle.
4. Call in the issue that requires healing between your hands, stating this three times and sign the Hon Sha Ze Sho Nen, Sei He Ki and Cho Ku Rei, then transfer your hands to the proxy, which in this case is the piece of paper.
5. Turn your attention to the left hand corner of the triangle and write the current issue, including all the people involved, the locale and situation, in point form. This area represents the current situation.
6. Now turn your attention to the right hand corner of the triangle and write your desired outcome, including the people involved and the locale.
7. The upper corner of the triangle is left blank, representing the Universal healing energy, power and protection – all the outer forces that would help in this situation.
8. Now begin your absent healing in the usual manner, calling in the issue in the standard manner.
9. Once the symbols have been signed and you have contact, transfer your hands to the proxy, which in this case is your paper in the lower left hand corner

(the current situation). Sign symbols intuitively and direct healing energy to the people and situation that is current. Send for approximately five minutes.

10. Now turn your attention to the lower right hand corner and sign any symbols needed and direct healing energy to the people concerned and situation for your ideal outcome. Send for five minutes.
11. Lastly, place your hands to the upper section of the triangle. Send healing energy to all those that would help.
12. Once you have finished, fold each corner into the centre. Firstly, the left hand corner to the centre, then the right hand corner to the centre and finally the upper corner to the centre. Here we bring all the elements together, combining and igniting this power. Hold this now between your hands for a short time until you feel it complete.
13. Now visualize the three symbols. Once you have completed this procedure blow through your hands and the folded paper three times to release the healing process.

You may choose to burn this mandala or keep it in a special place. In burning a healing triad, you symbolically release yourself from the situation and your attachments to the outcome.

Visualizing the Triad

This procedure can also be visualized by forming a triad with your hands, placing your thumbs and index fingers together to form a triangle. The person holds this mudra in front of them or over their own brow chakra, calling to mind the people and situations involved. The symbols are drawn with the tip of your nose and directed with your eyes. These can be blown with the breath into the areas required by following the procedure before.

Healing Triads on the body

This procedure can also be used on the body.

Whilst performing hands on healing, it is appropriate to use specific points on the body utilizing the same process. The left foot represents the left hand corner of the triad, the right foot represents the right hand corner of the triad and the heart chakra represents the top of the triad.

Here the facilitator signs a Cho Ku Rei for each corner, and follows the steps as before bringing all of these points together at the Hari of the individual signing the symbols on the body of the individual.

Healing Triads and Chakras

This process can also be used on one specific point or chakra of an individual. Once a chakra has been identified as requiring healing energy, then this chakra is the target of the process.

Here the facilitator places their hands on the chakra concerned forming a triad, with their thumbs and index fingers joined.

The Healing triad procedure is then visualized from this point to resolve the root cause of the issue determined from the life mapping process. This process can be repeated for subsequent chakras or other areas in need.

Chapter 17

'One single torch can dissipate the accumulated darkness of a thousand eons. Likewise, a single instant of clear light in mind eliminates the ignorance and obscurations accumulated over kalpas.'

— ***Tilopa***, Mahamudra of the Ganges

REIKI AND BUDDHISM

As is clear from Dr. Usui's original manuscripts, the origins of Reiki lie directly in the Tantra of the Lightning Flash, a teaching derived from early Buddhist traditions. With this in mind this next chapter is devoted to instilling some of the Buddhist methods of healing which combine some methods of Universal Reiki and Buddhist Tantra. It should also be noted that the methods presented here are not the actual practices which have recently been translated by Lama Yeshe, (notably Menchhos Reiki, Usui's Buddhist Reiki); rather these are simplified techniques which embrace some of the core teachings of the medicine Buddha tantra and other Tibetan healing practices. The methods presented offer the lay practitioner the opportunity to preview some of the introductory Buddhist practices and foundations in order to utilize these methods for the benefit of others.

The teachings presented here are methods for opening oneself to one's own awakened potential. One does not need to be Buddhist to practice these techniques, these methods open a practitioner to be able to generate positive results.

USING MANTRAS WITH REIKI

The use of Mantras holds particular frequencies for healing. The Mantras that are being referred to are the archetypal seed syllables for the vibration of Compassion and Healing. In the Buddhist tradition perhaps the most widely practiced mantra is: OM MANI PADME HUNG, the Buddha of Compassion 'Avalokiteshvara' (Sanskrit) or Buddha 'Chenrezigi' (Tibetan). The vibration of this mantra evokes the energy of unfolding compassion in the heart. Its essential meaning is "all praise to the unfolding of the jewel in the heart of the devoted". As with most mantras, it is important to receive where possible, the transmission of this empowerment from a qualified Lama (Buddhist Master or Geshe) in the form of a blessing 'Loung' or initiation 'Wonkur'. However, if this is not possible, then it is permissible to use these mantras with our Reiki or meditation practice and aim to at least receive this blessing and Buddhist refuge somewhere down the line.

The Buddha wants all beings to be free, regardless of position, belief or virtue. This is one of the reasons why the Buddhist teachings are given out of compassion for anyone who desires to learn.

To use a mantra is an experience of repeating these

syllables over and over, evoking the vibration and energetic maps they compose. Mantras can be sung, spoken slowly or quickly. It is best to explore which way feels appropriate for you.

Some popular Buddhist Mantras and their meanings:

OM MANI PADME HUNG

Buddha name: Avalokiteshvara.
Archetypal Deity: Buddha of Loving Kindness and Compassion.
Mantra translation: Om Jewel of unfolding Hung.

OM AMI DEWA HRIH

Buddha name: Amitabha.
Archetypal Deity: Buddha of Limitless Light, Guardian of Dewachen (Pure realm).
Mantra translation: Om Lord of Limitless Light Hrih.

OM TARE TUTTARE TURE SOHA

Buddha name: Green Tara.
Archetypal Deity: Buddha of Great Liberation.
Mantra translation: Om Liberitous, Liberate now.

OM DORJE SEMPA HUNG

Buddha name: Vajrasattva.
Archetypal Deity: Buddha of Purification (Diamond mind).
Mantra translation: Om Diamond Being Hung.

OM ARA PA CHA NA DHIH

Buddha name: Manjushri.
Archetypal Deity: Buddha of Wisdom.
Mantra translation: No translation literal in English. Mantra represents: 'Perfect Wisdom'.

OM GATE GATE PARAGATE PARASAMGATE BODHI SOHA

Buddha name: Prajinaparamita.
Archetypal Deity: Mother of all the Buddhas.
Mantra translation: Om gone, gone, gone completely beyond, awakening, let it happen.

TAYATA OM BHEKHANDZE BHEKHANDZE MAHA BHEKHANDZE BHEKHANDZE RANDZA SAMUNGATE SOHA

Buddha name: Sangle Mendela (Medicine Buddha).
Archetypal Deity: Buddha of Healing.
Mantra translation: Thus gone, healer, great healer King, accomplish healing, let it happen.

To receive empowerments for the various Buddhist archetypes contact your local Mahayana or Vajrayana Buddhist centre.

Out of the main branches of Buddhism there are three main traditions, these being the vehicles of Hinayana, Mahayana and Vajrayana. These empowerments are mostly prominent in the Mahayana and Vajrayana schools of Tibetan Buddhism. The best way of keeping informed of upcoming initiations for these archetypes is to be on the mailing lists or by attending meditation sessions at these centres.

BUDDHIST ARCHETYPES

Some of the Archetypes described previously, represent the vehicles of generating particular states of mind and their accomplishment.

The practice of these deities allows (particular to their use) the cultivation of certain positive qualities and the purification of obstacles. One should where possible, gain a deeper understanding from the caring guidance of a qualified lama. With right motivation, right understanding and the right methods, one can gain meaningful and lasting results.

MEDICINE BUDDHA, THE BUDDHA OF HEALING

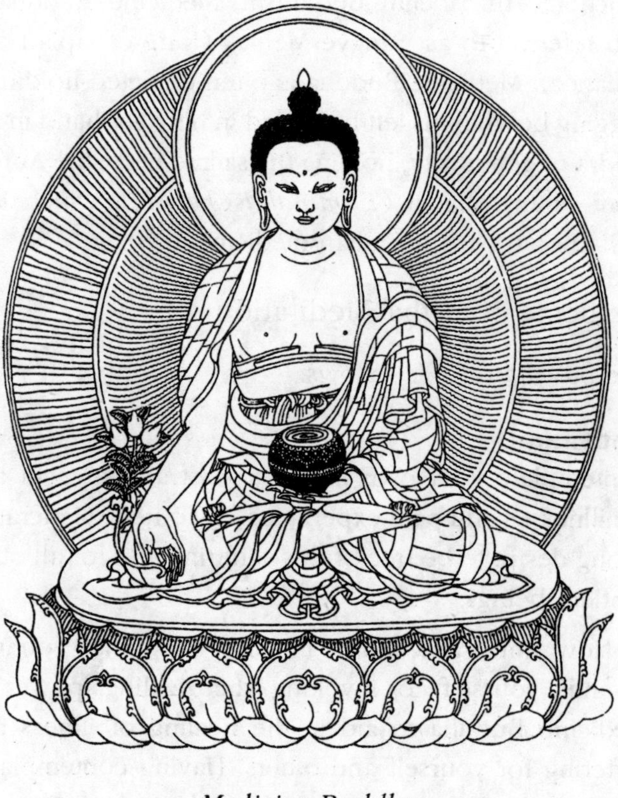

Medicine Buddha

Medicine Buddha is a Buddhist Archetype popular in Vajrayana Buddhist traditions. Medicine Buddha's practice is also very widespread throughout the Buddhist world. This practice has widespread popularity in Tibet, Nepal, Bhutan and Shingon Buddhist traditions. Medicine Buddha is depicted in the colour blue (Medicine Buddha's body), which in this practice represents the removal of physical disease, and a Gold robe, which represents the removal of mental, emotional and spiritual afflictions. In Tibetan Buddhism, Medicine Buddha is also referred to as 'Sangye Menla', (King of lapis lazuli radiance). Medicine Buddha is often depicted holding a begging bowl in his left hand and in his right hand in the mudra of generosity, holding the sacred herb, the Aurora plant or myrobalan (*Terminalia Chebula*); which is a well-known herb in Indian medicine.

Medicine Buddha Meditation

The procedure is as follows:

Motivation

Contemplate your own illnesses, past and present and the illnesses and pain experienced by others. Generate a strong desire to be free of this suffering and for all other sentient beings.

Now think and affirm in your mind that you will commit yourself to invoking the healing power of Medicine Buddha to aid in the healing of illness and suffering for yourself and others. Having contemplated these, we have set the ground of right motivation and proceed with the visualization.

The Visualization

Visualize Medicine Buddha either above the crown of your head or the crown of the person who you wish to bestow healing upon. The Buddha is a tenth of our size and faces the same direction as the recipient or ourselves.

He is sitting upon a lotus seat and moon coloured cushion. He is radiant, translucent blue in colour and his appearance is vibrant and beautiful. In his right hand he holds the Aurora plant in the mudra of supreme generosity. In his left hand is held a begging bowl, which is coloured blue with white inside, and contains medicinal nectar. This nectar is the ambrosia of life and all healing, containing all herbs, minerals, healing powers and forces beyond the physical realm.

Prayer of Request

I strongly request to you Medicine Buddha, please grant me your blessing, that I may completely purify my body, speech and mind and, thus, heal myself by developing my own innate Medicine Buddha nature.

I strongly request to you Medicine Buddha, please bestow your blessing upon me, that I may completely alleviate the suffering, both mental and physical, of every single sentient being.

Now imagine Medicine Buddha is delighted by your sincerity, prayers and requests and he emanates and radiates white light which pours from his heart, skin and begging bowl. This light pours like rain into our crown or the crown of another and completely fills the body and mind with this healing power. This light completely purifies all our disease, afflictions, mental obstructions, negative karma, emotional problems and negative feelings. See your body and mind becoming clear, clean and pure.

Whilst visualizing this purification, recite the Medicine Buddha mantra 21 or 108 times:

TAYATA OM BHEKHANDZE BHEKHANDZE MAHA BHEKHANDZE BHEKHANDZE RANDZA SAMUNGATE SOHA

Now imagine Medicine Buddha is emanating and radiates blue light which pours from his heart, skin and begging bowl. This light pours like rain and into our crown or the crown of another and completely fills the body and mind with this healing power. This blue light completely destroys all physical illness and disease and negative energies of the whole body. See your body becoming energized, strong and clear.

Whilst visualizing this transmission of energy and power, recite the Medicine Buddha mantra 21 or 108 times:

TAYATA OM BHEKHANDZE BHEKHANDZE MAHA BHEKHANDZE BHEKHANDZE RANDZA SAMUNGATE SOHA

Now imagine that Medicine Buddha reduces in size directly above our crowns to the size of a mustard seed. He enters the crown of our heads and travels down the central channel to our hearts. The Buddha dissolves into light and this light merges with our own body and fills us with light, healing and power.

Dedication

May the heart of awakening which has not yet risen,

arise now and grow. May that which has arisen never diminish, but increase more and more.

May the merit of this practice benefit all beings and may all beings be well and happy and free from suffering.

This completes the meditation.

Medicine Buddha and Absent Healing

Here we use guided imagery, the Medicine Buddha mantra, Reiki symbols and Absent healing to assist in the healing process for oneself or another.

Procedure

1. Call the person requiring healing by stating their name three times, and accessing their mind with the Sei He Ki. Once you feel a connection with the person, proceed with the following:
2. Draw: Hon Sha Ze Sho Nen, Sei He Ki, Cho Ku Rei.
3. Visualize Medicine Buddha above the recipient's head facing the same direction as them. Visualize white light emanating from Medicine Buddha pouring light rain and flowing into the body and mind of the recipient.
4. Whilst this is occurring, recite the Medicine Buddha mantra 21 or 108 times.
5. Now visualize a blue energy emanating from Medicine Buddha, which pours like rain into the recipient, energizing and clearing physical obstructions.
6. Whilst this is occurring, recite the Medicine Buddha mantra 21 or 108 times.
7. Once this is complete, visualize Medicine Buddha

condensing in space and travelling through the recipient's central channel, dissolving into the heart of the recipient, filling them with healing power and light.

8. Share the merit of this healing practice and give thanks in your own way.
9. Access to see if any further healing or mantras are required and place these in the Quantum healing bank to be accessed by the recipient at a later time.
10. Once this feels complete, draw: Hon Sha Ze Sho Nen, Sei He Ki, Cho Ku Rei.
11. Blow through cupped hands three times and seal your Thymus chakra.

This procedure can be extended by including the specific visualizations and details from the previous meditation on Medicine Buddha.

Medicine Buddha and Hands-on Healing

The healing qualities of Medicine Buddha can be incorporated into your hands on session in a similar fashion to your absent healing. Imagine or visualize a small Medicine Buddha above the head of the individual you are treating. The Buddha is facing the same direction as the recipient. As you are facilitating Reiki healing, see the streams of light coming from the heart of Medicine Buddha down through the crown chakra of the recipient and going to the affected areas, healing the obstructions that are causing illness and imbalance. As you are seeing this happen, all the while you are reciting the Mantra silently in your mind:

TAYATA OM BHEKHANDZE BHEKHANDZE MAHA BHEKHANDZE BHEKHANDZE RANDZA SAMUNGATE SOHA

Once you have finished the treatment, condense the Buddha into light and let it travel down the central channel where it resides in the heart of the recipient. Give thanks in your own way and finish in the usual manner.

In cases of serious illnesses do not dissolve the Medicine Buddha in the heart, rather see the Medicine Buddha continuing to radiate healing energy for the recipient.

This procedure can greatly increase the effectiveness of your sessions, while also receiving the Blessing, the bestowal of healing and merit from Medicine King Buddha.

The Importance of Direct Transmission

The complete empowerment for Medicine Buddha's teaching lies directly in the Menchhos Reiki system (Usui's Buddhist Reiki). The techniques described above are adaptations of a simplified form of this teaching.

For one to fully engage in the practices of Medicine Buddha, one requires the appropriate initiations from a Buddhist Lama. One also needs to take Refuge in the Buddhist teachings and receive the empowerments of the sacred texts concerning the practice. The form presented above acts as a starting point for all non-Buddhists and can be practiced by anyone who sincerely wishes to benefit all sentient beings with the healing power of Medicine Buddha.

These meditations can be adapted to your specific needs, you may want to visualize a fountain of light or an Angel or some other symbol that speaks to you. The symbolism we use is a tool to focus the mind on the practice.

I always encourage people to try a practice for a time and if this does not suit, then put it on the shelf and try something that does. These practices do take time and right effort, so it is good to work with these on an ongoing basis.

DEATH AND DYING

'Death is unimportant, Life is unimportant.
Life itself is a link in a chain or a ripple around
a rock in the flow of my stream.'
— Mikao Usui

BUDDHA AMITABHA, THE BUDDHA OF BOUNDLESS LIGHT

Assisting someone at the point of death can be a very empowering gift for the being making their transition as well as being a beneficial and personally liberating experience. Later in this chapter we will outline the methods which can assist an individual who has died, however there are certain factors which first need to be considered if we are to have a basic understanding of this process. Before we describe the practice in detail, it is important to outline some of the foundations from the Buddhist world view of what occurs in the death process.

What happens when we die?
Most of our familiar western (Christian) views on death are generally concerned with the lead up to one

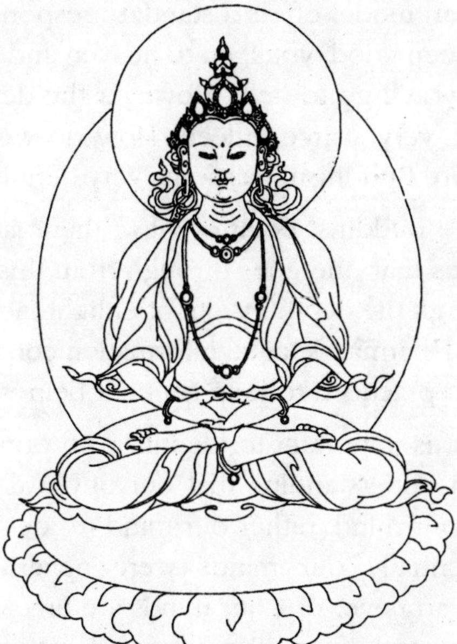

Buddha Amitabha

departure from this world with little consideration to the way one actually makes this transition. Usually if the person is religious, a priest is present to give the person confession and to say some prayers. Because Christianity has no system or concept of the inner channels, and instead relies heavily on faith and a belief in an outer force, once the person has died, it is largely a matter of hoping that the priest did a good job and that we will be met by a kind and forgiving God.

Essentially, with this model being belief based, the consideration of the internal workings of consciousness is largely left up to the Almighty to sort out. Often we asked as children, 'What happens to us when we die?'

The Christian model offers a standard response: 'Well, if you have been good, you'll go to heaven and if you have been bad, you'll go to hell.' However the details of this process are very scarce indeed. How do we get there? This is where Buddhism has some very definite answers.

From the Buddhist point of view, there is a certainty of the stages that one goes through from this life to our next. Through the depth insight of enlightened practitioners of the Dharma, detailed information concerning this transition is practiced to help sentient beings.

Firstly, it is important to identify with our minds and develop an understanding that our physical body does not create our mind, rather our mind resides within our body. Essentially our minds were never born, and therefore, can never die; our minds are timeless without beginning or end. If you like, our mind or true essence is like space, and our body is a vehicle or container for our mind during this lifetime.

Once our physical body ceases to function, our mind becomes once again like space, so wherever we think, then this is where we are. For example, we think of our loved ones and we are before them, we think of our favourite place in nature and there we are; the mind has no container (the body), and therefore can be anywhere at will. We know this is also true, with examples of how our thoughts shape reality. For example, when we think of a friend and the next day we bump into them or they call you on the telephone, and things like this.

The inner stages leading up to death and the stages that follow.

From the Tibetan Buddhist perspective there are essentially two phases of dissolution for someone dying. These are the outer dissolution, where the five elements or sense impressions dissolve or cease to function and the inner dissolution, where the inner channels, thoughts and emotions dissolve. So let us firstly look at the outer dissolution of a dying person.

As human beings we essentially are made up of five sense elements which are Earth, Water, Fire, Air and finally, Space which is our true essence or Clear Light.

In the moments leading up to one's death, the first of these senses to dissolve is the element of Earth. Here our body begins to loose all its strength, we are unable to hold ourselves upright, we feel heavy and uncomfortable in any position, we may ask to be propped up with pillows or for others to help us in keeping upright and stable. It becomes harder to keep our eyelids open and our mind becomes drowsy. This indicates the dissolution of the earth element.

The next element to cease functioning is the Water element. Here we lose control of our bodily fluids, our nose and eyes begin to run, we may dribble or even become incontinent.

Following this, the element of Fire begins to dissolve. Here we become very thirsty, our body begins to cool and the outer extremities become cold and lifeless. All of the warmth of our body begins to condense into the centre of the body and our minds swing between clarity and confusion. We find it hard to recognize loved ones as sight and sound are also confused. Our breath is cold as it passes through our mouth and nostrils and this leads us into the fourth element of Air.

As the Air element begins to dissolve, it becomes harder and harder to breathe. Our in-breaths become more and more shallow and our out-breaths become longer and longer. Our minds become a blur with no recognition of the outside world. Lastly we breathe out three long breaths and do not breathe in again, all our vital signs are gone and for all intents and purposes we are dead. Although this is when most loved ones pack to go home, from the Tibetan view, this is the beginning of the inner dissolution.

The dissolution of the inner winds

In the Buddhist perspective the dissolution of the inner winds takes anywhere from twenty to thirty minutes. The procedure that follows later in this chapter can be of particular benefit during this time, but more on this later.

It is during this time that the internal energies of the body collect in the central energy channel. It is at this point that the white energy that resides at the crown chakra which is eight finger-widths from the original hair line in the centre of the head, travels through the central channel from the crown to the heart centre. This process takes approximately ten to fifteen minutes. This White energy represents the Male or Sperm of the father essence. It is during this time that thirty three emotions related to anger are liberated.

Once this White energy reaches the heart centre, there is a tremendous light which is beyond words and beauty. The ecstatic sensation represents the liberation of the negative emotions relating to anger from the lifetime.

At this point, it is worth noting that in most research and case studies concerning N.D.E.s (near death experiences), we find a common element here. Often with N.D.E., the being is travelling through a white tunnel going to a tremendous light, and those who have come back to tell their tale describe the joy and renewed respect for life which come from such an experience.

This is also suggestive of the central channel, the liberation of negative emotions and our consciousness journeying along the central channel.

What follows next is the Red energy, representing the Female or egg of the Mother essence. This essence now begins to journey through the central channel. This Red essence resides in the navel, four finger-widths below the belly button in the centre of the body and comes up through the central channel towards the heart centre. This process also takes anywhere from ten to fifteen minutes and it is during this time that forty emotions relating to attachment are liberated. Once these two internal energies meet at the heart centre, the mind is like deep space. In this moment, seven emotions relating to Ignorance are liberated and with this there is an incredible light that is so overwhelming, the mind simply loses consciousness. This light is the true essence or clear light of our minds, but unless we are experienced meditators and can recognize this light as our own minds, the being loses consciousness for a period of anywhere between sixty eight hours to three or four days.

It is after this time that the mind of the being begins to wake up. Often the mind is confused from the experience and tries to communicate with friends and loved ones from the former life.

In the mind of the dead one, they perceive themselves as having a physical form. This is because the being is still strongly attached to their conditioned impressions from their former life.

As mentioned previously, the mind has no container (the body) and moves anywhere it senses as the thought arises in the mind.

Because the mind has no container yet it thinks it is still physical, the being will try to communicate with the living and receive no response. One will walk across fine sand and leave no prints, one will look into mirrors and see no reflection and eventually it dawns on the being that they are in fact dead. This is the intermediary state of the Bardo. It is during this period that experiences of friends or dear ones to the departed may experience that they can feel the deceased nearby, or that they are having a conversation with them. It is with these experiences that the being is making some contact on a psychic/telepathic connection to one's relatives or loved ones. Many people put this down to their imagination or wish fulfilment, but it is usually the case that contact is actually being made. This transitory state takes approximately seven days from the time of regaining consciousness. Once it dawns on the being that they must have died, the shock of this is so overwhelming that the mind slips once again into unconsciousness. It is then, through this time, that the strong subconscious impressions begin to surface. One will stay in these impressions till one has served out the necessary karma and then these impressions dissolve. This can last anywhere from a few hours or days and up to a total of forty nine days from the being's death. At this time a clear light comes and the being makes their transition from these Bardos to their next rebirth. In the transition to their next rebirth, one will see their future parents. Pulled by the Laws of Karma, the mind will go to the future parents, entering the male through the crown chakra during lovemaking. The consciousness is then born as the White male essence and Red female essence unites (sperm and egg in fertilization).

It is from here the being begins their next life and so it goes.

THE BLESSING OF THE PURE REALM, DEWACHEN

The procedure included can benefit a being to bypass these Bardos and go straight to a pure realm or a heavenly state (Dewachen). To assist one in this process, one needs to facilitate this under the following conditions:

- Between the point of death and the following thirty minutes.
- Between the third day to the forty ninth day of the person dying.
- This process can be facilitated either in the location of the deceased or as an absent healing procedure.
- This process can be continued till the seventh week or until there is no presence of the being at the calling in stage. (Stage 1 in the procedure which follows.)

Procedure to assist a being's transition through dying

1. Call the person in three times using the Absent healing procedure. If you are present with the individual, call in the mind in the same way. Once you have a clear sign that the mind of the individual is present, state briefly your intentions and what you will be doing for them. Remember, they have a psychic link to your mind at this point and know your thoughts, so this can either be said out loud or silently.
2. Sign the three symbols to bridge the Reiki energy to the one who has died: Hon Sha Ze Sho Nen, Sei He Ki, Cho Ku Rei.
3. Set your intention that there is a Red Buddha (Amitabha) above the head of the individual facing the same direction as they.
4. Now visualize the person going into the heart of this Red Buddha through the crown of their head and up through the body of Buddha Amitabha.
5. As you are visualizing this happening recite the Mantra 108 times, seeing them going into this Buddha. Recite: 'Om Ami Dewa Hrih'.
6. Recite three times the offering prayer: 'Buddha Amitabha, please bestow your blessings on 'state the being's name', and grant him/her/them the freedom from the attachment to this life, granting him/her/them the blessing of your pure realm, Dewachen.'
7. Repeat the visualization and mantras again or until you sense their movement from this world to the realm of Dewachen.
8. Once this feels complete, give thanks in your own way and dedicate the merit of this practice for the benefit of all sentient beings.

9. You may wish to offer your own prayers and set up additional Mantras and symbols in the Quantum healing bank for the individual.
10. Complete the healing by signing the three symbols: Hon Sha Ze Sho Nen, Sei He Ki, Cho Ku Rei and blow through your cupped hands three times.

In addition to this method, you may wish to send the idea to the person before they die, to think of going to the best thing they can think of directly above their heads, and to go to that when they die. One can also say the Mantra in the dying one's ear within the first 30 minutes after they have died, or say the Mantra over your fingers and place these on the crown of the individual's head. All these suggestions will assist in the transition of the individual, so they can bypass the often difficult transition between this world and the Bardo realms.

It should be noted that this procedure is a simplified form of Phowa and is not the actual and complete procedure. To perform Phowa, one requires specific instruction and the direct transmission from a qualified Buddhist Master (Lama). The method present here is an introduction to the concepts of assisting beings in their transition, and to confer a blessing and assistance in this process. It is highly recommended for one to accomplish a greater understanding of this process, that one completes a Phowa retreat, (conscious dying), with a qualified Lama as well as receiving Buddhist refuge and the initiation for Amitabha in the form of Wonkur (initiation).

For further reading on this subject and a deeper explanation of these concepts please refer to *The Tibetan Book of Living and Dying* by Sogyal Rinpoche.

BRINGING IT ALL TOGETHER

At this level the practitioner has worked with a large variety of ways of using the universal energy of Reiki. In one's Reiki practice, it is essential to consider each person that you treat in a new light each time. One can easily get into a routine of facilitating a Reiki session and doing the same techniques without consideration to the individual and their particular needs. Now this is fine if you are simply facilitating a basic Reiki I hands on treatment, the energy will work on a general level for that being's highest good.

If, however, you are working with specific methods for directing universal energy, i.e., directing symbols, Medicine Buddha, etc., your personal awareness, being centred and holding focus become vital factors in directing the Reiki energy in these specific ways.

To the best of our ability, our mind should be pure, with the aspiration of being a clear channel for the healing of Medicine Buddha and for this healing energy to be passed through ourselves and into the recipient. Treat your session much like a meditation, be watchful of your thoughts, watch your mind. If you feel yourself thinking about the weekend or what you are going to be doing later, then you are not there for the person, so bring yourself back and be watchful.

When we are present we are in flow in Body, Speech and Mind, and out of this comes the essence of being one with Reiki. It is good advice to cultivate this in your personal self-healing and in the treatment of others.

Chapter 18

'When you come to a fork in the road, take it.'

— ***Yogi Berra***

REIKI 3A

In this next Chapter we will attempt to illustrate some of the basic methods of the Third level. Not all of the methods are presented here, as these techniques require a readiness on behalf of the student and initiation into the third degree. One should only attempt to use the methods presented within this level, corresponding to your own level of initiation.

When it comes to the traditional Third degree in Reiki, the levels split into two sections, these are the A and B sides. The A side represents Practitioners and the B side represents Teacher training.

Although one can learn level 3A, and one is working with the power of the third degree, the A side does not qualify oneself as a Reiki teacher or as it is referred to in some Reiki schools, as a Reiki Master.

Teacher training or what could be referred to as Reiki Masters Training on the other hand, requires an additional initiation at this level and is further discussed in the next chapter.

The benefits of learning Reiki 3A are many. The following is an overview of what is covered during the training.

1. Participants receive the Reiki 3A initiation which gives them a huge increase in power and an ability to facilitate healing on much broader and expansive levels.

2. Participants receive the Reiki 3 Symbol which is the fourth symbol in the Reiki system, it is known in Amida Buddhism as 'The Great Light'. This symbol is used in the Reiki initiation procedures, which are taught to create a powerful alignment with the universal energy.

3. Participants learn a variety of advanced methods for local and non-local healing, including distant attunements, self-attunements, group attunements, healing locations, hands on initiation procedures, duplicating initiations and exploring various spiritual plains and methods of generating personal and spiritual power.

3. Participants learn the theory and practice of initiations, what they are and the keys to how they work.

4. In 3A, two initiations are imparted:

   A. The first initiation of Reiki I, which can be given to anyone and will give a temporary alignment to the Reiki energy. With this they can be shown the Reiki hand positions and start to use the Reiki on themselves. This initiation can also be given to someone who already has Reiki to greatly enhance their power.

B. The Reiki II booster initiation, which is given to people who are at least Reiki II or higher, to increase their power. It also may be sent over a distance to people, places, past and future.

WHAT THE 3A INITIATION ACHIEVES

The 3A initiation works on opening the inner ear and the divine eye which greatly increases the capacities of intuition, inner knowing, guidance and clairvoyance. It also works on the Solar plexus chakra by balancing issues of will, ego mind, personal power and issues of control.

The prerequisite for beginning 3A for advanced practitioners is a solid foundation in the practices of Reiki II and Advanced Reiki.

Here we begin to work with the initial steps of the Reiki attunement processes. This is said to be one of the most powerful levels, both energetically and spiritually, because here we are empowering others with Reiki.

Reiki I Temporary Alignment

This alignment gives the recipient the ability to empower themselves through hands on healing. This has proved most successful in clinical work, where the client comes for healing and wishes to continue their practice between sessions. This simple procedure transfers the Reiki energy, creating an alignment for the individual, so that they are taking an active role in their own healing process. This alignment has a temporary effect, the attunement lasts anywhere from three weeks to three months, these times vary from individual to individual.

SELF-ATTUNEMENT PROCEDURES

When bestowing self-attunements there are three methods to facilitate the Reiki attunements, and they are as follows:

Method 1. Physically drawing the Reiki I initiation procedure on oneself.

Here the student learns how to facilitate an attunement procedure on oneself. This is a valuable exercise to promote and activate the universal life force energy in daily life.

Giving self-attunements also boosts the immune system and acts as a means of purification and protection from negative influences.

Method 2. Completely visualizing the procedure.

This method is the same as the previous one, however it varies in the approach. Here the student uses creative visualization, there are a number of variations on this method, such as self-arising, front arising, third person and duplication methods.

Method 3. Visualizing and using mudra as symbolic memory cue.

Here the student combines these processes with a great emphasis on visualization. The method incorporates the use of mudra or hand gestures to determine where one is in the initiation procedure. These mudras also summon power and particular frequencies of the

Reiki energy and symbols. With practice, these mudras alone generate the power of the initiations.

Absent Initiations

Sending an Absent initiation is possible with any level of the Reiki system. The very notion that we can send Absent healing, makes Absent initiations only a step up to directing Universal Energy.

The procedure one follows is the same as Absent healing. Once the desired person is 'called in', their energy is transferred to a proxy of your choice. One then simply performs the initiation procedure, either physically, as if the individual were present, or by visualizing the procedure, using the law of correspondence to direct the attunement to the specific points of the energy system. One can also use one's own body as a proxy by performing a self-attunement procedure, corresponding this alignment to another. This way, both receive the initiation.

Another variation to this procedure is to have a photo of the person and to place this on a chair. Once the person has been called in, using the standard procedure, one performs the initiation process as if it were a person seated before them.

With all these approaches, it is important to close the procedure in a standard fashion as with Absent healing procedures.

Absent initiations can be particularly beneficial in assisting others during times when there is a great deal of negativity or suffering present within an individual.

This is also the case for particular locales, places or situations. Sending Absent initiations at a distance is a very powerful way to direct the healing power of Reiki to assist in the removal of negative forces and to aid in the best possible outcome of situations. In this way, the initiations align the individual, location, or object with the Reiki energy. This alignment has a powerful transformative effect.

Group Initiations

Aside from individual initiations, a number of students may initiate one individual at a time. This squares the energy and much like group hands on healing, there is a greater amount of Universal energy flooding the individual at one time. This has numerous effects for the recipient and can be used to remove strong blockages, obstacles, serious illnesses and negative patterns in the mind and emotional bodies.

The Great Light, Dai Koo Myo

DAI KOO MYO MEANING:

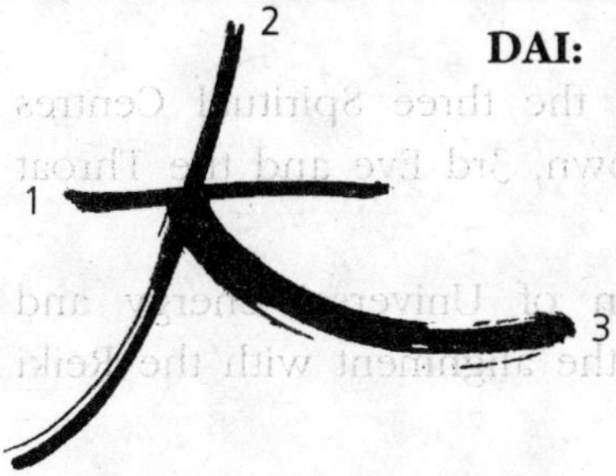

DAI: Big; huge; magnificent expansion; all-pervading.

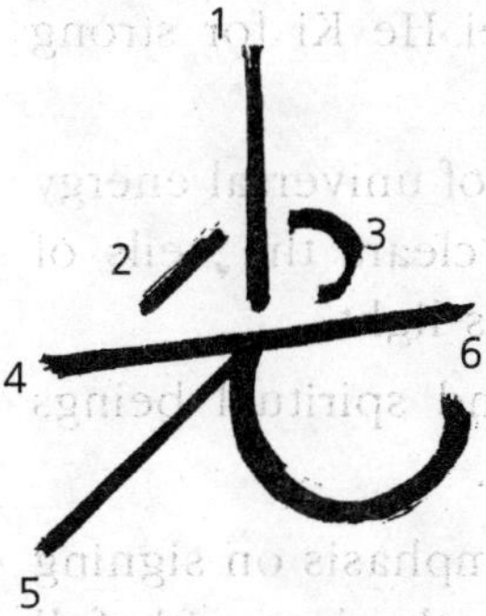

KOO: Light radiating in all directions; fine light; radiance; expansion at Crown Chakra.

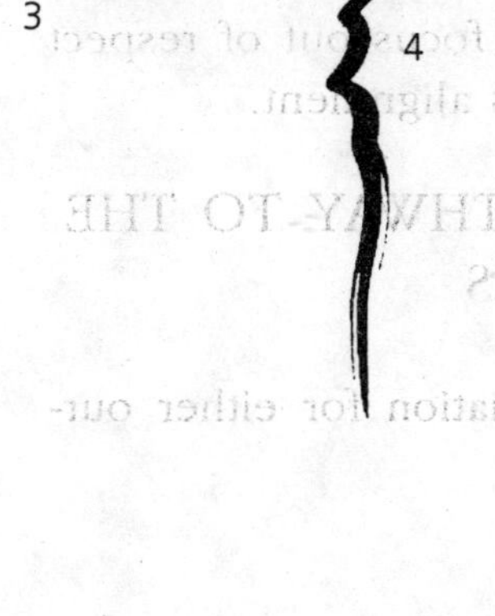

MYO: Too clear to doubt; clairvoyance; moonlight shining through the window; the divine light illuminating the darkness of ignorance; the merging of the sun and moon; forming a great light; the Enlightened One (the light of Buddha's wisdom, expansive all permeating light, radiating from the head (halo) of the enlightened one).

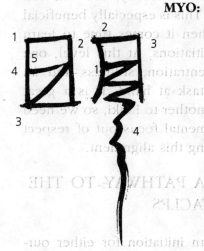

DAI KOO MYO USES:

- Dai Koo Myo activates all the chakras and energy channels.
- Dai Koo Myo affects the three Spiritual Centres above the Heart : Crown, 3rd Eye and the Throat Chakras.
- It activates the union of Universal energy and personal Ki, creating the alignment with the Reiki energy.
- Works in conjunction with Sei He Ki for strong protection and boundaries.
- Calls in a tremendous amount of universal energy which dispels negativity and clears the veils of ignorance that block the soul's light.
- It summons healing forces and spiritual beings who oversee the Reiki system.

As in Reiki II, there is strong emphasis on signing the Reiki Symbols not only correctly, but with full awareness and attention. This is especially beneficial training for the mind when it comes time to learn and perfect the Reiki initiations. At this level, one needs unshakable concentration, stillness and an ability to focus on the task at hand. It is a great responsibility to attune another to Reiki, so we need our full awareness and mental focus out of respect for the individual receiving this alignment.

REIKI INITIATION, A PATHWAY TO THE REMOVAL OF OBSTACLES

Each time we facilitate an initiation for either ourselves or another, we clear more and more of the veils that prevent our true inner knowing.

It is much like the analogy of the sun on a cloudy day. The sun represents ourselves, whole and awakened. The clouds represent our negative conditioning, ignorance, fear and delusion.

We all know the sun is there, but when the clouds are present we never actually see the sun clearly.

When we facilitate an initiation procedure, we are calling forth a tremendous amount of universal energy with the Dai Koo Myo and with each attunement procedure, we actively clear more and more of these clouds, thereby transforming ourselves in the process.

The initiation procedures are a great way to clear ourselves on a daily level. The practice of self-attunements or where possible, group attunements, gives participants the opportunity to refine their abilities of concentration and focus. These attunements also have subsequent purification and clearing which follows.

Some students facilitate the self-attunement procedures on a daily level, sometimes doing numerous attunements each day when working on specific issues.

One may say that one only needs to be attuned to the Reiki energy once, much like a doorway that has been unlocked. This is certainly true; however, the repetition of this practice clears the inner channels and energetic system of the body and subsequently has a direct effect on whatever requires healing or clearing within the body.

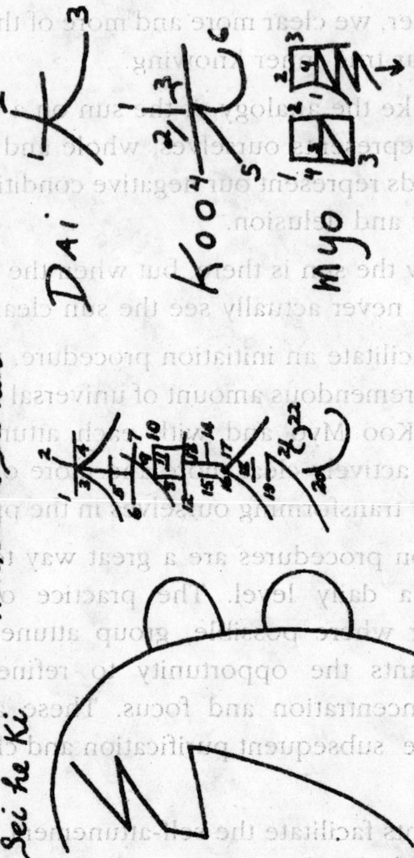

The 4 Reiki symbols
(Symbols kindly supplied by Independent Reiki Master, Gary Samer.)

MRS. TAKATA'S PERSONAL HANDWRITING OF THE REIKI SYMBOLS

Presented here are Mrs. Takata's personal handwriting of the Reiki symbols. As we sign and practice the Reiki symbols, it is suggested that both students and teachers use these examples as a source for emulating in their practice. Perfecting the form and working with these examples allows us to model Mrs. Takata's Reiki symbols, and as a result, have a close link to the source of the original Universal Reiki as taught by Mrs. Takata.

Chapter 19

'The most beautiful experience we can have is the mysterious. It is the fundamental emotion which stands at the cradle of true art and science. Whoever does not know it and can no longer marvel, is as good as dead, and his eyes are dimmed.'

— Albert Einstein

REIKI 3B TEACHER TRAINING PROGRAMME

The call, the decision to become a Reiki teacher

To become a Reiki teacher is a further step in one's path of service to humanity. Being a teacher of this system is not for everyone and requires a deep commitment to healing oneself and others.

If you like, to become a teacher is much like receiving the 'call'. The 'call' is found in many religious and esoteric traditions, a priest is called to the priesthood, a healer is called to the path of becoming a shaman or medicine person, and in many ways, a teacher of Reiki is called to teach. This is indeed an honour, and a privilege and should be considered carefully.

Being a Reiki teacher is to be a holder of the light. What this means is one who carries the Reiki lineage, the power of the Universal Energy itself and the responsibility to pass this on with integrity and honour.

Without these essential ingredients, one will falter. Ultimately, Reiki is a path of healing but more than this, it is a path of awakening. The more we actively embrace and live these practices the more our awakening and potential as human beings unfolds. That is Reiki as it should be.

Responding to this call, is not a matter of waking up one day and saying: 'I wonder what I'll do today. Oh, I'll become a Reiki teacher.' The call comes from a place deep within, it can certainly be activated by an experience in our lives, a chance meeting, an illness or relationship; it can simply be an inner knowing. However one comes to the decision to be a holder of the Reiki tradition, it is surely no small feat.

So in making the decision to become a teacher we need to consider our motivation very carefully; status, position and money should be at the bottom of your list. Candidates for teacher training are accepted with respect to understanding, practice and integration, personal motivation and integrity. The path of being a Reiki teacher is not necessarily an easy path, for it requires one to be a living example of Reiki and this means one needs to embody the practices and live Reiki to the best of our ability.

So here is an outline of the teacher's path and briefly what it takes to become a teacher.

Reiki 3B Teacher training is for those individuals who feel drawn to pass on the Reiki System. 3B takes the form of an apprenticeship and empowers the ability to permanently initiate and attune people to Reiki levels I and II. Participants learn workshop presentation and facilitation, initiation and attunement procedures.

The apprenticeship includes: co-teaching and participating in Reiki I and II workshops, coordination of Healing Clinics and related community service projects.

In addition to this, participants learn workshop presentation, personal development skills, group dynamics and other related spiritual disciplines which unfold throughout the training.

Participants also receive the 3B Initiation which empowers the person to teach Reiki levels I and II. The time duration for apprenticing varies from individual to individual. The training time is anywhere from nine months to two years. Teacher candidates are selected with consideration to personal development, previous experience, personal and spiritual integration and personal motivation.

The prerequisite to attending the training program is a completion of Reiki I, II, and Reiki 3A levels. A candidate of this level requires a direct lineage in the Reiki system and preferably, one should have received these initiations in sequence with the same Reiki teacher. This is to maintain consistency with initiation procedures, as their are many variations of these procedures from teacher to teacher.

Applicants are also required to submit a personal assessment life mapping questionnaire and an essay on why they wish to become a teacher of Reiki.

At the completion of the apprenticeship, the teacher in training participates in a three-day module to integrate the methods taught. At this point, final initiations are bestowed and the teacher is empowered to initiate students of their own in Reiki levels first and second degree. A new teacher may also continue to participate in workshops with the senior instructor to fine tune initiations and gain direct experience of being a teacher of Reiki.

Once a student has completed their training, they also receive a certificate in Reiki 3B and are granted the title 'Reiki Instructor' under the guidelines of the AIRT.

WHAT IS A REIKI MASTER?

This term was created when Reiki made its transition from the east to America in the early 1970s.

At the AIRT we do not refer to any teacher of any level as a Reiki Master.

Reiki is a path of humility and there is always more to learn.

Traditionally, in Japan, students could call a teacher 'Sensei' out of respect for their knowledge, an American Indian elder is called 'Grandfather or Grandmother' out of respect for their wisdom and status. Unfortunately, in the West we become infatuated with titles and position, often lacking in humility and respect.

The ultimate goal of any spiritual practice is to gain liberation from suffering and to benefit others in this goal. Self elation and ego inflation can be a real obstacle on the path and one needs to keep in check with this, or at least have friends or a spiritual teacher who has the kindness to burst your bubble.

The term Reiki Master was never actually used in Japan. It was adapted in the West for the purpose of position and power. We see today so many people pumping themselves up with titles to make themselves and their egos feel important.

There's a saying that goes: 'Anyone who says they are enlightened, isn't.'

One demonstrates their accomplishment through their actions of kindness and compassion.

It is through living Reiki, that we let our light shine for others to see. We should never encourage people to convert or recruit others into Reiki, it is only by example that others learn.

It would be foolish for ourselves to talk about how spiritual we are if we have not mastered our own minds. Therefore, it is essential to walk this path with deep respect and humility for the depth.

His Holiness the Dalai Lama puts this beautifully when he says that he is just a simple Buddhist monk. One should never put oneself above another or be beyond the basic tasks of life.

Humility is a virtue that is learnt with time. This is always why we give thanks for our lives and dedicate our newfound wisdom for the benefit of others.

FREQUENTLY ASKED QUESTIONS REGARDING TEACHER TRAINING

Q: *How long does it take to become a Reiki teacher?*

A: The length of time differs from person to person. At the AIRT we consider a candidate for teacher training after the person has been working with Reiki actively for at least a period of two years. The training time or apprenticeship can be anywhere from one to two years depending on the individual. This is in regard to teaching Reiki levels, first and second degree. The emphasis is on having a solid experience and understanding of the Reiki system. It would be foolish to give empowerments before a student is ready as they will not benefit nor integrate the wisdom of the teaching. So conversantly, the training that is offered is gradual, based on personal integration, humility and personal growth. To complete the full training takes much longer and is determined by the senior initiating instructor.

Q: *Is a Reiki Master more qualified than a Reiki teacher or Reiki Instructor?*

A: This is really a question of semantics. All these terms mean exactly the same thing. One does not become a 'Master' overnight, and really a grand title like this cannot be bought or sold. Mastery is something that is bestowed by one's students out of respect for their teacher. Unfortunately many people are calling themselves Reiki Masters to evoke grandeur and an ego-generated position within the spiritual scheme of things.

So, humility is an important consideration here. I would be very wary of someone who wanted to tell me, upon first meeting, that they were a Reiki Master, unless they were of white hair and supreme wisdom. Titles seem to evoke grandeur in people and are a subtle way to boost the ego-mind for one's self and position over others. Our egos are generally big enough without adding titles that put us above others and give ourselves the appearance of being highly sophisticated and special. An enlightened being does not need to advertise that they are enlightened.

Or, as the saying goes, if you meet the Buddha on the road, shoot him!

The Seminars

As part of the on-going mentorship and training, the Reiki Seminars are an excellent training ground for teachers in Training. A teacher-in-training may participate in several seminars as part of their training. The teacher-in-training's role is to at first observe and take personal notes on procedures, ask questions and to simply observe. One's ability to observe is an important part of becoming a teacher. It is through this method that one comes to learn group dynamics and the subtle group energies unfolding during a workshop.

After a teacher-in-training has a solid understanding of the techniques taught, there is then the opportunity to teach parts of the workshop and eventually co-teaching with the senior instructor. The time that this whole process takes varies from student to student and much is dependant on one's personal growth and integration of the level.

It is at the end of seminar participation where the student completes the final module of 3B.

Here the empowerment is given to 3B, the initiation procedures are taught for the four Reiki I empowerments and the Reiki II initiation. The teacher-in-training may also be asked to participate in a further two workshops after their 3B training module to assist the senior teacher in the initiation procedures of Reiki levels, first and second degree.

It is suggested that new Reiki teachers facilitate at least four Reiki I workshops before they facilitate a Reiki II workshop, or to wait at least a period of six months. The reasons for this are simple. It allows time to integrate the initiations of Reiki I. The new teacher needs this time to integrate, and this also allows the Reiki I students time before moving them to the second degree. Meanwhile, running other workshops and initiating others in first degree allows the teacher time to adjust to the higher frequencies running through his/her body. Naturally, it takes time to adjust to this level of the Reiki energy.

TEACHER TRAINING AND PERSONAL GROWTH

The Reiki 3B initiation and the teaching of Reiki levels brings up whatever issues are required for the teacher around personal power, self-worth and ego-mind. Like the other Reiki levels, 3B has a deeply purifying effect on the individual. With this in mind, some teachers consider or are made to consider their lifestyles and personal habits, as with this new level of empowerment, some habits, views and attitude simply do not mix with this level of the energy. Please refer to Dr. Usui's advice to his graduating students in Part One of this book.

BEING REALISTIC, BEING YOURSELF

It is surprising how many people develop a concept of being spiritual. This can be a trap of sorts, a way of replacing one set of neuroses with another. A common experience with personal growth is the misconceptions of the ego mind. What tends to go with this is a desire for all that is nice and good to stay and a neglect of the suffering and undesirable things of life. In denying our negative selves we can be out of balance. Naturally we all want to be free from suffering and learn to cultivate happiness. However, this cannot happen unless we are prepared to deal with our own shadow material. Self-acceptance is not about a single pointed idealistic view of ourselves. It is far better to accept ourselves from where we are.

When we experience pain or discomfort in our lives, our immediate response is to remove this discomfort and to change our current dilemma to more favourable situations. There are certainly many times when this is most appropriate; however, in facing and examining our response and even allowing ourselves to be still in that reaction can be a tremendous learning vehicle. The philosophy of being able to be still in the face of adversity and to move into that experience reveals much about our conditioning. So when someone presses your buttons either through careless words or actions, instead of reacting to this, try to identify the cause of the reaction. People are our mirrors, be watchful and you begin to see yourself.

Power, Ego and Reality Checking

Because level 3B works specifically on the solar plexus chakra, issues relating to self identity and personal power often emerge as a result of this empowerment.

As we further our understanding in the practices and methods of this level, students often experience ego, with a capital 'E'. The overall effect of the 3B initiation affects the solar plexus and as a result, any latent issue to do with our ego comes to the surface. This is seen as a positive cleansing of these issues; however, it is important to know how to deal with these issues when they arise.

One direct way to awaken humility is to take the attention off, 'What's in it for me?', and instead, earnestly generate compassion for all that lives.

The following are some suggestions for keeping a lid on our egos:

1. Ask for others' feedback in your teaching abilities and how you interact with others.
2. Look at your response when others give you criticism.
3. Keep a journal of your positive responses to Reiki

and look at your personal motive for being a teacher.

4. Be prepared to look at your shadow issues and seek outside guidance when needed.
5. Dedicate, daily, all your actions, abilities, belongings, your body and mind for the benefit of all that lives.
6. Donate a part of your earnings to a worthy cause, give donations to charities, offer service to others and give some of your time away without the expectation of return.
7. Write a list of your short-comings, now compare these with your personal attributes.
8. Daily, offer prayers that all beings be well and happy and free from harm.
9. Surrender to the movement of spirit in your life. Let go, let spirit guide you.
10. Have purpose to your day, live each day dedicated to love and awakmening.

Discount Teacher Training

In recent years, Reiki has been making some significant changes on an international level. Some of these changes have unfortunately included the commercialization of Reiki as a marketable product.

Like many great eastern traditions as they make their way to the West, a certain amount of dilution and complexity occurs. Today it is possible to obtain all Reiki levels in a one-day workshop for a suspiciously low fee.

This of course heeds no reference to the traditional system, nor does it honour one's personal and spiritual development. If we look at this issue through the eyes of common sense, we see that in fact, Reiki is an ongoing practice which takes years of time and practice to distil the inner awakening that each level potentially bestows to the sincere student.

The following article, written by myself, addresses some of my personal concerns regarding how Reiki is being offered today.

Quality Control

In the West today, Reiki is taught in a variety of forms and has grown at an exponential rate. Skimming through any new age mag, it's easy to become baffled by all the 'Reikis' available, ranging not only in content and the speed at which one can learn, but also in price – part of the ever-growing new age consumer supermarket. It seems, with so many healing modalities 'out there', you can become enlightened almost instantly, or perhaps led astray? The Reiki system has in many ways become misrepresented in translating the system from its former roots in Japan. With such an enthusiastic response the world over, quality control in training of teachers has become a big issue. To attain a correct and pure alignment with the Reiki energy, it requires an unbroken lineage of teachers who are qualified and empowered to pass on the Reiki System. It is for this reason one cannot learn Reiki out of a book, or just become a Reiki practitioner or Reiki Master (teacher) overnight. Like most spiritual traditions, integration and practice plays a big part in embodying and understanding this healing art. Similarly, if we use the analogy of mastery in martial arts, one does not become a black belt, without practice, experience and a deep understanding of the principles involved. This is equally the case for becoming a teacher of Reiki. Unfortunately, in our consumer society we can so easily be sold the 'quick fix'.

Traditional Reiki is an exact science of energy renewal. This connection is engendered through a series of attunements, with each attunement building on subsequent levels. Once each level is embodied and one has an understanding, both spiritually and experientially, one is then ready to extend the connection to further levels.

This is often, or should be regarded as, a gradual process under the guidance of a qualified and reputable Reiki instructor. Having said this, there have been many arguments to counter these ideas, views that are often fixated on vague idealism without consideration to the practicalities of personal growth.

Today, many people are proclaiming to be 'Reiki Masters', many the result of a one-day workshop. Titles like 'master' often breed a sense of exclusiveness and spiritual elitism in many people and it is often not till later in one's journey, that one learns; humility plays a big part in embodying the teacher levels. This is in no way intended to disrespect the legitimate teachers of the traditional Reiki system, however, it should be stated that Reiki Mastery is not only an honour, but a life-long pursuit.

So what does one look for in a legitimate teacher of this system? It is hard to know who has the goods merely from an advertisement in the paper. We find that most Reiki teachers state that their Reiki is the traditional original Usui System. So how can the practice of a single system have so many anomalies and variations and still be under the same banner? In truth, not all Reiki systems are the same. To achieve the alignment to this energy in its purest form requires an unbroken lineage of teachers who have not only the correct Reiki symbols and initiation sequences, but the empowerment from their teacher in the true lineage.

It seems that people are getting a little wiser these days and asking more questions before they invest their time, money and most importantly, their spiritual lives. But alas, as it is with many systems of healing there will no doubt always be a few cowboys, blazing new and uncharted trails and boldly going where no one has gone before!

To summarize, being a teacher of Reiki requires a deep responsibility and personal integrity. This is because, as teachers we are not only shaping our own lives, but the spiritual lives of others. We would be wise to make sure the ripples of our pond don't make tidal waves. Ultimately we all have our lessons to learn, but a wise choice is better served by an educated one.

Teacher Training Requirements

The following is the AIRT 3B training candidates' information and application. This is designed to map out the commitments required and personal self-evaluation necessary in taking such a step. This self-assessment process is an interesting process in itself. It is designed to take a deep look at your genuine desire to begin the training. Often this process is very illuminating with regard to one's shadow and accessing one's authentic self.

The Reiki Teachers Training programme is an apprenticeship offered by the Australian Institute for Reiki Training.

In undertaking such a commitment there are a number of requirements to be satisfied.

The following endeavours to highlight these requirements and what it means to embark on the path of Reiki Teachers Training.

The commitments in this path are broken down into three parts:

1. Your first commitment is to Spirit, the Universal energy and the way in which this shapes your life.
2. Your second commitment is to your own healing process and the pursuit of the path of healing others.
3. Your third commitment is to the Reiki Lineage, the teachings and the teachers of the tradition.

The role we take in passing on this modality offers tremendous personal and spiritual unfoldment as well as the responsibility of being a living example of the path. As you begin this journey you will find the universal energy shaping you and readying you as a vessel for universal energy. This translates as a purification and healing of our personal agendas.

As we deepen our commitment, we begin to recognize the inner wisdom of Reiki. This in itself is hard to convey in words. The result of being in the energy and especially in having the responsibility of teaching and initiating others brings with it many gifts. We become closer to the source of our own becoming. There is a deep understanding of peace, humility and awareness. Becoming a teacher does not mean that you will become more spiritual, rather you are shown the door. The stepping through, is the practice, dedication and embracing the teachings.

As a teacher, we hold the keys of an exact science to awakening. This is not only a great honour, it is a way of life. Our aim is to embrace our greatness and remember our humanness. As seekers of the path, we recognize our foibles and take the challenge to move beyond to something far greater.

The AIRT Teachers Code

As teachers of Reiki we should endeavour to honour the teachers code.

1. All AIRT Reiki Instructors acknowledge, honour and respect Mikao Usui as the founding father of Reiki.
2. AIRT Reiki Instructors acknowledge all other legitimate Reiki schools and teachers, regardless of personal differences and beliefs.
3. AIRT Reiki Instructors agree to a uniform and consistent approach with regard to initiation, methodology and practice.
4. AIRT Reiki Instructors strive for personal and professional excellence as representatives of the standards and ethics of the AIRT.

AIRT Teachers Training

The AIRT teachers training for Reiki 3B takes place progressively over time and as part of an apprenticeship. This culminates as a three-day module upon completion of the training to integrate all that has been learnt. The AIRT aims for a standard of excellence in facilitation, personal integrity and professionalism in the teaching of the Reiki system.

Prerequisites for 3B

1. A sincere desire to serve humanity in the pursuit of healing, personal integrity and active compassion.
2. Your preparedness to support and to be available for your initiating teacher and your fellow students.
3. Your willingness to understand, integrate and learn the material in the training programme.
4. An openness to practicality, grounding and humour in your approach to learning.
5. The completion and submission of your personal life mapping assessment questionnaire.
6. The completion and submission of your essay of personal motivation for teachers training.
7. The completion of Reiki levels I, II, Advanced, and 3A.
8. A personal commitment to upholding the standards and ethics held by the AIRT.
9. An acceptance of the AIRT Teachers training code.
10. The completion and submission of the application for AIRT teachers training.

Progressive training prior to completion of 3B

- Participating, co-teaching and assisting in Reiki workshops.
- Demonstrating an ability to organize, coordinate and promote Reiki workshops, clinics and related promotional events.
- Showing an active interest in participating in Reiki clinics, support groups, personal healing, personal practice and other related projects.
- A willingness to donate time and energy to service those in need and to community based services.
- Serving an apprenticeship and spending time with the Initiating Reiki Instructor.

A teacher in training is required to have met the standards necessary held by the AIRT. Completion of the training and final initiation is determined by the initiating Senior Reiki Instructor. When the teacher-in-training is seen to have gained this level of competency, the final training module is set. The time frame for teacher-training is of the personal discernment of the initiating instructor.

PERSONAL LIFE MAPPING ASSESSMENT

QUESTIONNAIRE
(Parts A and B to be submitted prior to the commencement of the training.)

Part A

Answer these questions as best as you can. This is an exercise for you.

1. In the past, what have I realized in the areas of...
   - Family?
   - Work?
   - Friendships?
   - Relationships?
   - Spiritual Path?
   - My Shadow?
   - Personal Growth?
2. What have I wanted but never had in these areas?
3. What brings me out of harmony in relation to...

   A. My path?

   B. Myself?
4. What are my greatest fears in relation to....

   A. My path?

   B. Myself?
5. What roles do I play in my life? Which of these serve my path?
6. What do I need to do right now to further my journey along my path?
7. What are my strengths? What are my weaknesses?
8. What is my definition of myself as a teacher of Reiki?
9. What is my purpose in this life? How can I fulfil this purpose?

Part B
Essay (approximately 1000 words).

Write as honestly and authentically as-you-know-how, warts and all!

'Why do I want to be a Reiki Instructor and what does this mean to me?'

Chapter 20

'Knowing all things, having experienced all things, and having developed that compassion which in any situation does not waver, but stretches onward until it is perfected in the supreme Buddha Mind.'

— ***Mikao Usui***

ADVANCED TEACHER TRAINING LEVELS

Senior Reiki Instructor

At the AIRT, a teacher who has completed their teacher training and has been upholding the tradition, teaching and practices of Reiki can request the Initiation of Senior Reiki Instructor. A teacher may also be invited by a Senior Instructor to receive this level of Initiation. Generally, this level of initiation is only offered after an instructor has been actively teaching for a minimum period of two years. This level of empowerment allows a teacher to initiate a teacher. It makes sense then, that for this to occur, one needs a solid experience in teaching to have the authority in making another a teacher. It would be unwise to initiate another as a teacher without the necessary personal experience.

The following is an outline of Senior Reiki Instructor Level.

This level of teacher's training, empowers the individual to initiate and train a student to be a teacher. This then enables the teacher in training to teach levels I and II in the Western Reiki System.

A teacher who has completed the Senior Instructor degree is empowered to teach Reiki levels: I, II, 3A, and 3B training programs and seminars. This level requires a long standing commitment to the Reiki system. The candidate is required to have been actively teaching Reiki I and II seminars successfully for at least a period of two years.

The teacher in training covers initiation procedures for the higher levels and facilitation of 3A and 3B training seminars. In addition to this, there are a variety of personal and spiritual practices which uphold throughout the training. Upon successful completion of the training with the initiating Senior Reiki Instructor, the candidate is then empowered to teach and receives a certificate and is granted the title 'Senior Reiki Instructor'.

About the Australian Institute for Reiki Training

The Australian Institute for Reiki Training was born out of the need to preserve professional standards in the teaching and practice of Reiki. Through the AIRT, students have the opportunity to receive training in Reiki by accredited facilitators who are of a professional standard.

Equally, recipients of this modality can be sure that a treatment from an AIRT Reiki practitioner will provide a service of quality standards.

At the institute, we strive to present teaching that is creative, informative and innovative, yet also holds true to the historical tradition, ethics and practice of the Reiki system.

Part of the vision of the AIRT is to offer training that bridges the differences between cultures, methodology and tradition.

In this way the AIRT sees its place by maintaining quality to the community at large, and healing for those in need.

The AIRT Mission Statement

The Australian Institute for Reiki Training is dedicated to the pursuit of healing, education and personal/spiritual empowerment for individuals and the community by maintaining professional standards and integrity in teaching and facilitation of the traditional Reiki System.

The AIRT Code of Ethics

1. AIRT practitioners shall conduct themselves in a professional and ethical manner, perform only those services for which they are qualified, and represent their education, certification, professional affiliations and other qualifications honestly. AIRT practitioners do not in anyway profess to practice medicine, psychotherapy or related practices, unless licensed to do so.
2. AIRT practitioners shall maintain clear and honest communications with their clients, and keep all client information, whether medical or personal, strictly confidential.
3. AIRT practitioners shall discuss any problem areas that may contravene the use of Reiki, and refer

clients to appropriate medical or psychological professionals when indicated.

4. AIRT practitioners shall respect the client's physical/emotional state, and shall not abuse clients through actions, words or silence, nor take advantage of the therapeutic relationship. AIRT practitioners shall in no way participate in sexual activity with a client. They consider the client's comfort zone for touch and for degree of pressure, and honour the client's requests as much as possible within personal, professional and ethical limits. They acknowledge the inherent worth and individuality of each person and therefore do not unjustly discriminate against clients and fellow Reiki practitioners.

5. AIRT practitioners shall refrain from the abuse of alcohol and drugs. These substances should not be used at all during professional activities.

6. AIRT practitioners shall strive for professional excellence through regular assessment, personal development and by continued education and training.

7. Equality is practiced with all AIRT practitioners, regardless of which level, (including teachers/instructors), within the institute and related practices.

8. AIRT shall honour all other recognized and legitimate Reiki systems, practitioners and teachers regardless of personal differences and beliefs.

9. AIRT practitioners shall refrain from making false claims regarding potential benefits of Universal Reiki.

10. AIRT practitioners shall in no way endeavour, either

by personal act, word or deed to bring the AIRT or its teachers and tradition into disrepute.

Reiki at Work in the Community, Reiki Healing Clinics

Reiki Healing Clinic

The Reiki healing clinics offer a formal ground to actively contribute healing within the community. Some of the ways the healing clinics benefit are as follows:

- A practice ground for Reiki students to hone their skills.
- A low cost service to the community from competent practitioners.
- The ongoing education and promotion of Reiki and its benefits to humanity.
- The clinics give the general public an opportunity to experience Reiki, and to ask questions before they invest time and money into a course.
- The clinics assist in generating positive energy, healing, moral and ethical standards as well as contributing to peace and healing throughout the community.
- Students can develop their abilities and are mentored by senior practitioners.

So far the Reiki Institute has participated in establishing several Reiki clinics in urban & rural areas, for cancer patients, and for special interest groups in the spiritual and alternative arena.

Reiki, a Look to the Future

The practice of Reiki has made tremendous movements in the West for over 20 years and has seen a great deal of change and expansion in a variety of forms. From the historical discoveries of Dr. Usui's notes and teachings, to the new Reiki styles and healing systems which have emerged from the original teachings, and in so many other ways.

The essential factor in all of this is healing. In a modern world, with so many stresses on the environment and in personal and spiritual lives, Reiki in its essence remains a healing power of beauty, simplicity and unconditional love. Where it will take us is unknown, however, one thing is certain, and that is the ongoing exploration of Reiki. With our innate curiosity as human beings, we can only move a further step forward to the great mystery.

> *'There are three steps to contentment: Love another, be loved by another, and love what you do.'*
>
> — ***Lawrence Ellyard***

Epilogue

Stepping on the path.

As a teacher of this system, I am often asked how I began my spiritual journey. My response is that I received a parking ticket. Now as strange as this sounds, it was this action which ignited a decision in my life. One day I had to run an errand and through careless thinking, I parked my car on the wrong side of the road, facing the wrong direction. Subsequently, I received a parking ticket. As I was feeling the financial pinch at the time, the parking fine was tremendously aggravating. At this time of my life, with my career in hand, I began to question why. I was having doubts about my career which, for many years had meant the world to me. 'Is this what my life is all about?'

Suddenly I realized, my car was my vehicle, the way I was moving from one place to another and ultimately through life. As I was facing the wrong way, down the wrong road, it dawned on me that I was facing the wrong path and I needed an immediate about-face. Some days later, I met my Reiki teacher and everything fell into place. It was upon this meeting that I knew this would be my vocation, my path. It was frightening and exciting. I stepped forward and Reiki embraced me.

Bibliography

The Reiki Factor, Second Edition, Barbara Ray, Ph.D., 1986, Radiance Associates, St. Petersburg, Florida.

*The Breath of Awakening, A guide to liberation through Anapanasati Mindfulness of Breathing,*Namgyal Rinpoche, 1992, Bodhi Publishing, Kinmount, Ontario.

Pranic Healing, Choa Kok Sui, 1990, Samuel Weiser, INC York Beach, Maine.

Healing Secrets throughout the Ages; Second Edition, Catherine Ponder, 1985, Devorss Publications.

Traditional Reiki for our times, Amy Z. Rowland, 1998, Healing Arts Press Rochester, Vermont.

The Tibetan Book of Living and Dying, Sogyal Rinpoche, 1992, Rider Books, London.

Essential Reiki, A complete guide to an Ancient Healing Art, Diane Stein, 1995, The Crossing Press Inc., Freedom, CA.

Hands of Light, A guide to healing through the Human Energy Field, Barbara Ann Brennan 1988, Bantam Book.

Reiki, the essential guide to the ancient healing art, Chris and Penny Parkes, 1998, Vermillion London.

Reiki, Penelope Quest, 1999, Piatkus, London.

Reiki, The Healing Touch, First and Second Degree Manual, Revised and Expanded Edition, William Lee Rand, 1998, Vision Publications.

Reiki Fire, Frank Arjava Petter, 1997, Lotus Light Publications, Shangri-La.

Reiki, the Legacy of Dr. Usui, Frank Arjava Petter, 1998, Lotus Light Publications, Shangri-La.

Reiki, Way of the Heart, Walter Lubeck, 1996, Lotus Light Publications, Shangri-La.

The Dhammapada. 1997 Element.

Native Healer, Initiation into an ancient art, Medicine Grizzlybear Lake, 1991, Quest Books.

Australian Flower Essences for the 21st Century, Vasudeva and Kadambii Barnao, 1997, Australasian Flower Essence Academy, Perth, Australia.

The Mirror of Mindfulness, The cycle of the Four Bardos, Tsele Natsok Rangdrol, 1987, Shambahala, Boston.

The Jewel Ornament of Liberation, The Wish-fulfilling Gem of the Noble Teachings, Translated by Khenpo Konchog Gyaltsen Rinpoche, 1998, Snow Lion Publications Ithaca, New York.

Luminous Mind, the Way of the Buddha, Kalu Rinpoche, 1997, Wisdom Publications, Boston.

The Good Heart, His Holiness the Dalai Lama, 1996, Rider Books, London.

Buddhism, Flammarion Iconographic Guides, Louis Frederic, 1995, Flammarion Paris-New York.

Vessantara, Meeting the Buddhas, A guide to Buddhas, Bodhisattvas and Tantric Deities, Tony Mcmahon, 1993, Windhorse Publications.

The Womb, Karma and Transcendence, A Journey towards Liberation, Namgyal Rinpoche, 1996, Bodhi Publishing, Kinmount, Ontario.

Shingon Esoteric Buddhism, A Handbook for Followers, Abbot Yusei Arai, 1997, Rt. Rev. Iwatsubo Shinko, Director, Department of Education of Koyasan Shingon Mission (Kongobuji).

Personal Medicine, Dr. Ralph Locke, Ph.D., 2000, SCI Publication, Chapel Hill, North Carolina.

Menchhos Reiki, An Introduction to the Secret Inner Practices, Venerable Lama Yeshe, 2000, FULL CIRCLE Publications, New Delhi, India.

Practising Reiki, Jennie Austin, 1999, Geddes and Grosset, UK.

Everyday Enlightenment, Dan Millman, 1998, A Hodder and Stoughton Book.

Reference Manuals

The Reiki Alliance Manual. Paul Mitchell 1985. Reiki Alliance.

Traditional Japanese Reiki as taught by David King and the TJR website.

Reiki III Reiki Master Course with Brian and Carole Daxter, 1993.

The Official Reiki Handbook, The official Reiki Program. A complete Reference Manual for students of Reiki. Barbara Ray, Ph.D., 1983.

Newlife Reiki Seichim and Newlife Seichim Manuals. Living Light Energy. Margot 'Deepa' Slater 1991.

Newlife Reiki Master Teacher Training with Margot 'Deepa' Salter, 1995.

A Japanese Reiki article published in Japan in 1986.

'Iyashi No Te', by Toshitaka Mochizuki, 1995.

'History of Japanese Religion', by Masaharu Anesaki, 1963.

'Shingon, Japanese Esoteric Buddhism', by Taiko Yamasaki, 1988.

The life story of Mikaomi Usui, by Gejong Palmo, Master of Reiki. 1997, the Way of Reiki.

Notes and Thoughts on the Buddhist Connections with Reiki, by Gordon and Dorothy Bell, Reiki Teachers. United Kingdom.

History of the Lightning Flash Tantra, Ven. Lama Yeshe, Menchhos Reiki.

Medicine Buddha Sadhana, thanks and appreciation to: Ven. Zasep Tulku Rinpoche, Ven. Geshe Sonam Rinchen, Ven. Jampa Gendun.

Glossary

Abbot: The principle or head teacher of a monastery in Buddhist traditions.

Amida Buddha: see Amitabha.

Amitabha Buddha: (Sanskrit) The Buddha of boundless light and boundless love. Among the five Buddha families, he belongs to the padma or lotus family and resides in the pure realm of Dewachen.

Aurora: (Sanskrit) The medicinal herb held in the right hand of Medicine Buddha, symbolizing healing. Also a common herb used in Indian Ayurvedic medicine.

Avalokiteshvara: (Sanskrit) The Buddha of compassion, love and kindness. Among the Bodhisattvas, Avalokiteshavara is perhaps the most venerated Buddhist deity.

Baihui: An acu-point found on the top of the head, the Baihui is the governing acupuncture point and is the location of the crown chakra.

Bardo: (Tibetan) The state between two other states of being. In particular the intermediate state between one life and the next.

Bodhidharma: (Sanskrit) Bodhidharma is a semi-mythical figure, mainly worshipped by the Chan and Zen sects. In Japan he is called Nanakorobi Yaoki (seven falls, eight recoveries), because according to tradition, Bodhidharma claimed that a follower struck down seven times will rise again an eighth time, thus, demonstrating that one cannot strike down a firmly established spirit. The number eight is a symbol of infinity and stability in Japan.

Bodhisattva: (Sanskrit) A key religious concept of Mahayana Buddhism. A Bodhisattva, having developed compassion for all sentient beings, is a person who is on the way to perfecting their own Buddha nature. Thus, he or she has dedicated his or her life to the well-being of others, having vowed to lead all sentient beings to complete liberation. This term also describes particular Buddhist Deities who assist sentient beings from their suffering.

Bodhisattva Vow The compassionate wish to forgo enlightenment till all beings are liberated from Samsara.

Bonze: (Japanese) A title for a teacher or master of eastern spiritual traditions.

Buddha: Literally, 'the awakened one'. One who has attained Supreme Enlightenment; the embodiment of all virtues and perfection. Also the name of the historical Buddha, the spiritual teacher, Gautama Sakyamuni (c500B.C.)

Burdurya Probassa Buddha: (Sanskrit) Another name for Medicine Buddha. Literally, 'the Buddha of Lapis Lazuli Radiance'. See Medicine King Buddha.

Chakra: (Sanskrit) Wheel, centre, eye, energy nexii within the subtle energy body.

Chenrezigi: (Tibetan) The Buddha of compassion. He is the patron and protector of Tibet and also a meditation deity, whose practice is very widespread, Tibetans believe that all successive Dalai Lamas are human manifestations of this deity.

Chi Kung: A Chinese style of energy work involving stances, visualization, breath work and slow Tai Chi - like movements to cultivate a balance of elemental energies in the body for health and long life.

Confucius: A Chinese philosopher whose teachings are popular throughout Asia.

Daimyo: (Japanese) A Lord or Noble, a title for one who holds land and title.

Dalai Lama: Literally 'ocean of wisdom' is the title given to the supreme authority of Tibet. The lineage of the Dalai Lamas has continued without interruption up to the present fourteenth holder of this title: His Holiness Tenzin Gyatso, born in July 1935. The Dalai Lamas are emanations of Chenrezigi, the Buddha of compassion, who is the patron and protector of Tibet.

Darwinism: Refers to Charles Darwin (1860) whose teachings and theories state: that the origin and perpetuation of new species of animals and plants of a given organism vary. That natural selection favours the survival of some of these variations over others, and that new species have arisen and may continue to arise by these processes. In broad terms: biological evolution.

Dewachen: A pure land or realm of Buddha Amitabha and Chenrezigi. The practices and wishes with them direct the mind at the time of death to be reborn there, liberated from samsara.

Dharma: (Sanskrit) Derived from the etymological root meaning 'to hold', Dharma denotes the teachings of the Buddha, the 'truth' or the 'way', and the practice of those teachings. The Dharma holds us back from suffering and its causes. The Tibetan equivalent 'Chhos' literally means 'change' or 'transformation' and refers to both the process of spiritual transformation and the transformed result.

Fudo Bodhisattva: (Japanese) A wrathful protector deity in esoteric Shingon Buddhism. In Sanskrit, his name means 'Immovable Radiant King'.

Gaijin: (Japanese) A derogative term used to describe westerner or outsiders in 19th century Japan.

Geshe: (Tibetan) A term to describe a monk who has attained a high level of accomplishment in doctrinal learning and has had many years of monastic education. Its literal meaning is 'spiritual friend'.

Giri: (Japanese) Giri is best described as: 'obligation', 'vow', 'debt'. To honour agreements made, to repay good deeds, to speak well of another, if one has acted or spoken well in return. To do these acts is said to have and to accumulate 'Giri'.

Guru: (Sanskrit) A title to represent a spiritual teacher and mentor of high accomplishment, who has unshakable spiritual virtue and wisdom. The minimum qualities a guru must possess are compassion towards student, inner discipline, a degree of serenity, and more knowledge on the subject that is being taught than is possessed by the student.

Hamachiman Bodhisattva: (Japanese) The Japanese God of War, who was converted to Buddhism by Kobo Daishi.

Hara: (Sanskirt) Refers to the energy centre situated just below the navel. Also referred to as the Sacral Chakra, is associated with the seat of personal power and vital life force.

Hari: (Japanese) The Japanese equivalent to Hara.

Hinayana: (Sanskrit) Literally meaning 'lesser vehicle'. One of the three levels of Buddhism, its emphasis is on purification and individual liberation, which acts as a foundation for the other two levels, Mahayana and Vajrayana. The Hinayana Buddhist tradition is most prominent in the southern schools of Buddhism, namely Sri Lanka, Thailand, Burma, Cambodia, Indonesia and Vietnam.

Honen: (AD 1133-1212) The name of the spiritual master who founded the Jodo-Shin sect in Japan during the Kamakura period (AD 1185-1333).

Kalpa: (Sanskrit) Generically, an aeon or other nearly limitless length of time. In Buddhist cosmology, it has the specific meaning of a complete cycle of a universe (a mahakalpa or 'great' kalpa consisting of four stages: emptiness, formation, maintenance, and destruction. Each of the four stages consists of twenty intermediate kalpas (antahkalpas), each of which increases and declines.

Kami: (Japanese) Used as an adjective in ancient Japanese to refer to anything mysterious or sacred. These subjects range from simple objects of folk cults to the deities of cult clans. Kamis may be deities of nature, controlling certain natural phenomena or locals, conceptual deities, embodying certain values, ideals or sentiments, or the protective deities of a clan.

Kanji: The Japanese word for Japanese pictographs or writings.

Kannon: (Japanese) The Japanese name for Quan Yin (Chinese) or Avalokitesvara (Sanskrit), the archetypal deity of mercy and compassion. Generally taking on a gentle, female form, Kannon is understood to protect living beings with loving compassion. According to the Avalokitesvara sutra, Kannon has thirty-three different forms. The most fundamental forms of these many manifestations are the seven Avalokitesvaras, which include: the Sacred, the Eleven Faced, the Thousand Armed, the Wish Fulfilling, the Horse Headed, the Mother Goddess and Avalokitesvara with rope and net. Each manifestation serves humanity in many individual expressions and is a popular tradition for most of Asia.

Karma: (Sanskrit) Karma refers to an important metaphysical concept related to action and its consequences. Literally meaning, 'action'. Whether these are physical, verbal or mental acts they imprint habitual tendencies in the mind. Upon meeting with suitable conditions, these habits ripen and manifest in the future.

Kobo Daishi: (AD 774-835) The name of the spiritual master who founded Shingon Buddhism in Japan.

Ksitigarbha Bodhisattva: (Sanskrit) The name of this Bodhisattva means: 'He who encompasses the earth'. Often depicted in six forms, each form is responsible for the six Paths of Transmigration: hells, hungry ghosts, beasts, demons, human beings and heavenly beings. Each emanation vows to save people from sufferings and disasters. The vows and protective amulets of Ksitigarbha lend power to those who are vulnerable, such as children..

Kundhyo Massage: A traditional Japanese form of bodywork.

Kwannon: (Japanese) The Japanese name for Quan Yin or Avalokitesvara.

Lama: (Tibetan) See Guru.

Lao Tzu: (300 BC) A famous Chinese sage who wrote the 'Tao Te Ching', the first classic teachings of the philosophy of Taoism.

Mahavairochana: (Sanskrit) Mahavairochana, literally means: 'Great Illuminator'. In Shingon Buddhism, he is the main deity of worship. Mahavairochana is the great solar Buddha of truth and light. His teaching accordingly corresponds to the 'first turning of the Wheel of the Law' by the historical Buddha. He is a personification of the Absolute.

Mahayana: (Sanskrit) The 'great way' or 'great vehicle'. Those schools of Buddhism that teach the Bodhisattva ideal — of selfless striving to gain enlightenment so as to be in the best possible position to help all other living beings to be released from Samsara.

Manjushri: The Buddha of wisdom. His name means 'The Bodhisattva of Beautiful Splendour'. He is traditionally depicted wielding the sword of wisdom with his right arm while in the left he holds the stem of a lotus flower on which rests the Perfection of Wisdom Sutra.

Mantra: a string of sound-symbols recited to concentrate and protect the mind. Many Buddhist figures have mantras associated with them; through reciting their mantra one deepens one's connection with the aspect of Enlightenment which the figure embodies.

Medicine King Buddha: In Sanskrit his name means 'the Buddha of the Master of Medicine'. Medicine Buddha is the governing deity of Usui's Reiki tradition and the Tantra of the Lightning Flash. Medicine Buddha (Yakushi Nyorai, in Japan) is the Buddha who offers medicine to beings suffering from illness, and grants nourishment to the mind and body. As a Buddha who carries out the functions of a physician among a large number of Buddha's, he holds a medicine container in his left hand. In his right hand is held the Aurora herb with his hand held in the mudra of granting vows. Medicine Buddha is perhaps one of the most important deities to the Japanese Reiki system.

Menchhos Reiki: The name given by the Ven. Lama Yeshe to describe Dr. Usui's original Reiki system. Literally: 'Medicine Dharma Reiki'.

Meridians: A term to describe the energetic channels of the body.

Merit Storehouse: The accumulation of any virtuous thought or activity that has the result of imprinting positive habitual tendencies in one's mind stream.

Mudra: (Sanskrit) Describes movement, gesture, seal, stamp, impression. Usually refers to specific positions of the fingers or gestures, each signifying a particular aspect of dharma; also dance postures and positions of the whole body.

Nicherin: (AD 1222-1282) The name of the spiritual master who founded the Nicherin sect in Japan during the Kamakura period (AD 1185-1333). The primary path of Nicherinism is the attainment of Buddhahood by chanting the Lotus Sutra.

Nirvana: (Sanskrit) Literally: 'extinction', to cease, to blow, to extinguish. That dharma which remains after complete craving has been eradicated; the emancipation from all sorrows; extinction of all roots of unwholesomeness, namely, greed, hatred and delusion.

Pali: The language of Northern India in which the Buddha taught; subsequently used to transmit and preserve the teachings; later written, i.e., The Pali Canon.

Phowa: A High Tantric practice of Vajrayana Buddhism. The ejection of consciousness to a Buddha-field at the moment of death. Also referred to as 'Conscious Dying'.

Prajnaparamita: The 'Perfection of Wisdom', direct intuitive insight into the true nature of things, through which one overcomes ignorance and thereby the principle of suffering. In Tantric Buddhism it is also the name of a female deity who is the embodiment of the Perfection of Wisdom.

Ratnagarbha: The first known successor of the 'Tantra of the Lightning Flash', as taught from Shakyamuni Buddha. His name literally means: 'Womb of Jewels'.

Refuge: Describes One's confidence in the precious ones, the three jewels: The Buddha, Dharma, and Sangha.

Sadhu: A traditional name for a holy man. Typically, in Hinduism, an ascetic who dedicates his life to spiritual self mortification, often performing daily spiritual practices of an extreme nature, in aid of purifying the body and mind.

Sama Bodhisattva: (Sanskrit: Samantabhadra) His name means the Bodhisattva of Universal Beauty. He represents the Buddhist Law and compassion, often associated with Manjusri Bodhisattva. He is also the protector of the Lotus Sutra and mainly worshipped bv the Tendai and Shingon sects.

Samsara: (Sanskrit) Literally: 'perpetual wandering'; the uncontrolled cycle of birth and death in which sentient beings driven by unwholesome actions and conflicting emotions repeatedly perpetuate their own suffering. Cyclic existence.

Samurai: A military retainer of a Japanese daimyo practicing the chivalric code of Bushido, a warrior of aristocracy of Japan.

Sangha: (Sanskrit) The term Sangha refers to the community of practitioners of the Buddhist path. As one of the three Refuges, it refers to the Arya or Noble Sangha, those Buddhist practitioners who have gained insight into the true nature of things and whose progress towards Buddhahood is certain. In other contexts the term can refer to those who have taken ordination as Buddhist monks or nuns.

Sangle Mendela: See Medicine King Buddha.

Sanskrit: Describes the ancient Indic language that is the classical language of India.

Sensei: A term to describe a teacher of Traditional healing, Martial or Spiritual arts.

Shakyamuni Buddha: The 'sage of the Shakyans', an epithet of Gautama Siddhartha, the founder of Buddhism.

Shiatsu: A Japanese form of massage, as a complete system of healing through touch, drawing extensively on key aspects of traditional Chinese medicine. A nurturing massage promoting health by influencing the body's natural flow of energy via the energy pathways known as meridians.

Shingon: Established in Japan during the Heian period (AD 794-1185) by the spiritual master Kodo Dashi. The path of Shingon is to realize Buddhahood in this very life, to dedicate to the wellness and happiness of all beings and to establish the world of Buddha on earth. The word Shingon literally means: 'true words' and refers that the teachings are based on the words of the Buddha.

Shogun: (Japanese) One of a line of military governors ruling Japan until the revolution of AD 1867-68.

Sutra: (Sanskrit) (from the same root as sota, to hear). The written discourses of Buddha Shakyamuni, constituting all the teachings.

Tabis: The Japanese name for footwear common in Usui's day.

Tai Chi: Popular throughout Asia, Tai Chi consists of slow flowing movements that follow a set pattern. Often linked to martial arts.

Tantra: Literally: 'thread'; Vajrayana teachings outlining mystic practices as the most direct way to enlightenment. A form of Buddhism making use of yogic practices of visualization, mantra, mudra, and mandalas, as well as symbolic ritual, and meditations that work with subtle psychophysical energies. Also the Buddhist texts in which these practices are described.

Tendai: The name of the Sect which formed in Japan during the Heian period (AD 794-1185). Tendai was founded by Saicho (AD 767-822) Formal title: Dengyo Dashi. The path of Tendai is to attain Buddhahood through the practice of chanting sutra, meditation, precepts and esoteric Buddhism.

Transpersonal: Extending or going beyond the personal or individual. Also describes a movement of modern psychology derived from Jungian Psychology.

Tulku: (Tibetan) Literally: 'Emanation Body'. A tulku is a reincarnate Lama; that is, one who has been formally recognized as the reincarnation of his or her predecessor. A tulku has the ability to direct their next rebirth.

Vajrasattva: (Sanskrit) A Buddhist Tantric archetype of purification. Literally: 'Diamond Being'; a being of utter purity dwelling in the complete union of wisdom with the skill and means to awaken this in others.

Vajrayana: (Sanskrit) Literally: 'Diamond Vehicle'; the instantaneous, direct path of awakening and transcending all duality. One of the three levels of Buddhism, it is distinguished by its variety of practices to bring a being quickly to liberation.

Wa: (Japanese) A Japanese word which represents harmony, balance, community, and peace.

Wei-To Bodhisattva: (Japanese) The Japanese and Chinese version of the Tibetan deity Vajrapani.

Wonkur: (Tibetan) Empowerment Transmission. An initiation in which a specific enlightened mind-energy-body state is invoked by the Lama and transmitted to the student.

Yakushi Nyoria: (Japanese) See Medicine King Buddha.

Zen: (Japanese) A school of Mahayana Buddhism found mainly in Japan and Korea. 'Zen' is derived from the Sanskrit word 'dhyana', meaning meditation and Zen places great emphasis on the practice of seated meditation. It aims not to rely on words and logical concepts for communicating the Dharma, often preferring to employ action or paradoxes.

Contact Details

If you, the reader, would like to contact the author please write to:

The Australian Institute for Reiki Training,
C/o PO Box 548 Fremantle Western Australia 6959.

Email: lawrence@webace.com.au
reiki@ozzienet.net

Or

Visit our International Reiki Institute website online at:
www.taoofreiki.com

Or

The official International Medicine Dharma Reiki website at:
www.medicinedharmareiki.com